Patrick Holford BSc, DipION, FBANT, NTCRP is a leading spokesman on nutrition in the media, specialising in the field of mental health. He is author of over 30 books, translated into more than 20 languages and selling over a million copies worldwide, including the *Optimum Nutrition Bible* and *Optimum Nutrition for the Mind*.

Patrick Holford started his academic career in the field of psychology. In 1984 he founded the Institute for Optimum Nutrition (ION), an independent educational charity, and was involved in groundbreaking research showing that multivitamins can increase children's IQ scores – research that was published in the *Lancet* and was the subject of a *Horizon* documentary in the 1980s. He was one of the first promoters of the importance of zinc, antioxidants, essential fats, low–GL diets and homocysteine-lowering B vitamins such as folic acid.

He is chief executive of the Food for the Brain Foundation and director of the Brain Bio Centre, the Foundation's treatment centre. He is also an honorary fellow of the British Association of Applied Nutrition and Nutritional Therapy, and a member of the Nutrition Therapy Council.

Also by Patrick Holford

100% Health
500 Top Health and Nutrition Questions Answered
Balance Your Hormones (with Kate Neil)
Boost Your Immune System (with Jennifer Meek)
Food GLorious Food (with Fiona McDonald Joyce)
Hidden Food Allergies (with Dr James Braly)
How to Quit Without Feeling S**t (with David Miller and
Dr James Braly)
Improve Your Digestion
Natural Chill Highs
Natural Energy Highs
Natural Highs (with Dr Hyla Cass)
Optimum Nutrition Before, During and After Pregnancy
(with Susannah Lawson)
Optimum Nutrition for the Mind
Optimum Nutrition for Your Child (with Deborah Colson)
Optimum Nutrition for Your Child's Mind (with Deborah Colson)
Optimum Nutrition Made Easy
Say No to Arthritis
Say No to Cancer
Say No to Heart Disease
Six Weeks to Superhealth
Smart Food for Smart Kids (with Fiona McDonald Joyce)
Solve Your Skin Problems (with Natalie Savona)
The Alzheimer's Prevention Plan (with Shane Heaton
and Deborah Colson)
The Fatburner Diet
The H Factor (with Dr James Braly)
The Holford 9-day Liver Detox (with Fiona McDonald Joyce)
The Holford Diet GL Counter
The Low-GL Diet Cookbook (with Fiona McDonald Joyce)
The Little Book of Optimum Nutrition
The Low-GL Diet Bible
The Optimum Nutrition Bible
The Optimum Nutrition Cookbook (with Judy Ridgway)
The 10 Secrets of 100% Healthy People

patrick
HOLFORD

BEAT
STRESS
AND
FATIGUE

THE DRUG-FREE GUIDE TO
DE-STRESSING AND RAISING
YOUR ENERGY LEVELS

piatkus

PIATKUS

First published in Great Britain in 1999 by Piatkus
Reprinted 2000 (twice), 2001, 2003, 2004 (twice), 2005, 2006, 2007, 2009
This edition published 2010

A CIP catalogue record for this book
is available from the British Library.

ISBN 978-0-7499-5358-4

Edited by Kelly Davis
Designed by Paul Saunders

Typeset by Phoenix Photosetting, Chatham, Kent
Printed and bound in Great Britain by CPI Mackays, Chatham, Kent

Papers used by Piatkus are natural, renewable and recyclable
products sourced from well-managed forests and certified
in accordance with the rules of the Forest Stewardship Council.

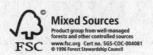

Mixed Sources
Product group from well-managed
forests and other controlled sources
www.fsc.org Cert no. SGS-COC-004081
© 1996 Forest Stewardship Council

FSC

Piatkus
An imprint of
Little, Brown Book Group
100 Victoria Embankment
London EC4Y 0DY

An Hachette UK Company
www.hachette.co.uk

www.piatkus.co.uk

CONTENTS

ACKNOWLEDGEMENTS

Writing a book on stress and fatigue could be very stressful and tiring. Not so, thanks to many people who have helped me tremendously. These include Natalie Savona, Rachel Winning and Kelly Davis. Also thanks to Dr Jeffrey Bland and his colleagues for their great work on unravelling detoxification and its role in chronic fatigue syndrome, to Susie Clift for her help on sleep research, and to the Arica Institute and Siddha Yoga for everything I've learned beyond nutrition.

Guide to Abbreviations and Measures

1 gram (g) = 1000 milligrams (mg) = 1,000,000 micrograms (mcg or μg). Most vitamins are measured in milligrams or micrograms. Vitamins A, D and E are also measured in International Units (iu), a measurement designed to standardise the different forms of these vitamins which have different potencies.

1mcg of retinol (1mcg RE) = 3.3iu of vitamin A (RE = Retinol Equivalents)
1mcg RE of beta-carotene = 6mcg of beta-carotene
100iu of vitamin D = 2.5mcg   100iu of vitamin E = 67mg
1 pound (lb) = 16 ounces (oz)   2.2 lb = 1 kilogram (kg)
1 pint = 0.6 litres   1.76 pints = 1 litre
In this book calories means kilocalories (kcal)
2 teaspoons (tsp) = 1 dessertspoon (dsp)
1.5 dessertspoons = 1 tablespoon (tbsp)

References and Further Sources of Information

Hundreds of references from respected scientific literature have been used in writing this book. Details of specific studies referred to are listed on pages 153–154. More details on most of these studies can be found on the internet for those wishing to dig deeper. PubMed is a service of the US National Library of Medicine that includes over 18 million citations dating back to 1948. This is where you can access most of the studies mentioned (see http://www.ncbi.nlm.nih.gov/pubmed/). On page 155 you will find a list of books to read to follow up information in this book.

DISCLAIMER

Although all the nutrients and dietary changes referred to in this book have been proven safe, those seeking help for specific medical conditions are advised to consult a qualified nutrition therapist, clinical nutritionist, doctor, or equivalent health professional. The recommendations given in this book are solely intended as education and information, and should not be taken as medical advice. Neither the author nor the publisher accept liability for readers who choose to self-prescribe.

All supplements should be kept out of reach of infants and children.

INTRODUCTION

CHAPTER 1

THE PRIMATE'S GUIDE TO 21ST-CENTURY LIVING

Being healthy means having a sense of well-being, characterised by a consistently high level of energy, emotional balance, a sharp mind and ability to cope with stress. Feeling tired a lot of the time, or spending most of the day stressed out with a knot in your stomach, is not healthy.

This poor state of being has become, for many of us, the norm. It's something we live with. Our performance may be somewhat blunted, the spark in our life somewhat dim, but we get on with it. At the other end of the scale are those with chronic fatigue who can barely function, let alone hold down a job, or those who are so stressed out that life is a permanent roller-coaster.

But this stress and fatigue syndrome, whether mild or severe, can be cured. To do so we need to gain a whole new understanding of ourselves: how our bodies make energy; how we respond to stress; the nature of our minds; how we have evolved to need certain chemicals or nutrients; and why others can throw everything out of balance. In short, stress and fatigue are signs that a person is having difficulty adapting to the myriad changes – nutritional, chemical, physical, social and psychological – that make up modern living.

OUR CHEMICAL HISTORY

Consider for a moment the chemical history of human beings. For three million years we were hunter/gatherers, eating all our food raw. Then, for ten thousand years, we were peasant farmers, eating whole organic food. Then, wham! – the industrial revolution and the birth of the modern, refined, processed, high-fat, high-sugar, high-meat diet. In the 1990s the American Chemical Society registers its ten-millionth man-made chemical (3500 of which are in our food and 3000 of which are in household products, from toiletries to cleaning materials). Then there are pollutants, pesticides and water contaminants. The result is that the average person's blood now contains 2000 chemicals that the evolution of *Homo sapiens* has never previously exposed us to.

OUR PHYSICAL HISTORY

Human beings have spent the past three million years being very physically active. We even have a 'fifth gear', triggered by the release of adrenalin. This boosts the efficiency of our muscles by increasing our fuel supply (in the form of blood sugar) and improving delivery of oxygen (the fire that lights the fuel). For our ancestors, stress required a physical response – to fight or take flight from predators.

Today stress is induced by pressure at work, traffic jams, financial problems, family rows, or watching thriller movies. What physical response do these 'threats' require? How do our bodies cope with all the chemicals released in a state of stress, chemicals that are designed to be burned off by exercise?

Modern man expends a fraction of the physical energy of his ancestors, and many of us aren't even fit enough to do a push-up or sit-up. We live in a push-button world where almost every physical activity has been replaced by an energy-saving gadget. But whose energy is it saving? Is the technology serving us or are we serving it? There's an old Chinese proverb, 'He who chops wood gets warm twice.' So how can we redesign our physical lives to promote health and energy, and truly use technology to give us a better life?

OUR PSYCHOLOGICAL HISTORY

On a social and psychological level, the world has changed beyond all recognition. Only three generations ago, a person's life presented two major decisions: who to marry and what profession to follow. Today marriages last, on average, three years. Many people move from one relationship to another, with all the stresses of separations and new beginnings. The same is true of work, with ever-decreasing job security. Ironically, when our standard of living should be going up, many of us are working harder than ever before, with less leisure time, while others suffer the stress of unemployment. The rapid pace of new technologies means that we have to keep learning new skills just to stand still. It isn't unusual to wake up with one's mind racing with an endless 'to do' list and to spend most of the day with one's thoughts spinning like a carousel. As one psychologist pointed out, 'We have over 6000 thoughts in a day and most of them are repeats.'

Some of us are good at adapting and everything is fine. But some of us are not. Our ability to adapt partly depends on having fully functioning immune, nervous and endocrine (hormonal) systems. Is it any coincidence that hormonal problems, such as infertility, breast and prostate cancer and menopausal problems, are increasing? That mental health problems – from depression and anxiety to schizophrenia – now affect one in six people in Britain? That Alzheimer's is reaching epidemic proportions? That 'chronic fatigue syndrome', allergies and the incidence of inflammatory health problems, from asthma to eczema, are increasing rapidly in children and adults alike? At the very least, this manifests as a lack of energy, poor concentration and memory, feeling tired all the time, depression and inability to cope with stress. These are all signs of mal-adaptation.

But this book isn't all doom and gloom and anti-technology. Quite the opposite. The 21st century requires new and better ways to communicate, organise and act for a better world. So how can we adjust our diet and lifestyle in order to survive and thrive in the 21st century? How much more could you expect from yourself if you had a consistent, high level of energy, emotional balance, a sharp mind and memory, and the ability to fight off every winter bug and cope with the inevitable stresses of life?

These are the questions my colleagues and I, at the Institute for Optimum Nutrition, have been exploring for many years. We've tested our ideas out on 30,000 people and now feel well qualified to say that there is an answer to stress and fatigue. It requires a change of mind, and a change of body – or, at least, what you put into it.

MIND AND BODY

It's not surprising that if you fundamentally change what you put into your body you will fundamentally change how you think and feel. After all, consider alcohol. One drink can change your mood and thinking, affecting both your behaviour and your level of physical tension. This link led us to explore whether changing a person's nutritional intake could increase their intelligence. Our experiments back in the 1980s proved that giving people optimal amounts of vitamins and minerals increased their IQ scores.

Further research showed that people didn't get cleverer as such. In tests their actual ability to solve problems wasn't much improved. What did change was the speed at which they solved problems. The change in IQ scores seems to be the result of faster mental processing, improved concentration and longer attention span.

Other studies have shown that changing a person's nutrition improves their mood. In a survey conducted by the Institute for Optimum Nutrition, which involved giving people 'optimum nutrition achieved with dietary changes plus supplements', 79 per cent noticed an improvement in energy, 60 per cent had better memory and mental alertness, and 66 per cent felt more emotionally balanced.

Over half (54 per cent), had previously rated high on a simple stress check (shown below), scoring five or more 'yes' answers. After six months on optimum nutrition the number with a high stress rating had dropped to only 28 per cent. Simple nutritional changes almost halved the number of high stress scorers. Yet these questions had nothing to do with nutrition.

Test Your Stress

Answer the questions below, ticking those that you answer 'yes' to.

☐ Is your energy level lower now than it used to be?

☐ Do you feel guilty when relaxing?

☐ Do you have a persistent need to achieve?

☐ Are you unclear about your goals in life?

☐ Are you especially competitive?

☐ Do you work harder than most people?

☐ Do you easily become angry?

☐ Do you often do two or three tasks simultaneously?

☐ Do you get impatient if people or things hold you up?

☐ Do you have difficulty getting to sleep?

All this illustrates that what you put into your body has a very powerful effect on your energy level and your ability to adapt to and cope with stress, on a mental, emotional, physical and chemical level.

THE CHEMICALS OF COMMUNICATION

To cope with stress, your body has to keep the right balance in the chemicals of communication whose job is to keep you 'well tuned' and functioning at peak level. These chemicals (primarily hormones, neurotransmitters and immune cells, about which you will learn more in later chapters) are made from the food you eat. If you don't have the right supply, your communication network starts to break down. Imagine your body as a city, with all its different residents, businesses, trading activities, communication and delivery networks. If there's a shortage of essentials, or a strike on a transport system, nothing runs smoothly. Everything slows down. Stress levels rise.

This is what happens to us when our total input – nutritional, environmental, psychological, physical – doesn't meet our needs or exceeds our ability to adapt. The symptoms are stress and fatigue. The following chapters put this jigsaw puzzle together. Certain pieces of the jigsaw will be more important for some people, than for others. However, somewhere in this book you will find the key pieces that will help you to improve your vitality and sense of well-being.

CHAPTER 2

THE VICIOUS CIRCLE OF STRESS AND FATIGUE

Most of us are sub-optimally nourished. This means that our body cells cannot make energy efficiently, so the first sign of sub-optimum nutrition is fatigue. This is nothing new. Throughout history, fatigue and stress have existed and man has searched for ways to conquer both. This has led to the use of 'stimulants' (or chemicals that give you a boost) such as tea, coffee, cigarettes, chocolate and sugar.

Stimulants boost your energy levels by stimulating your adrenal glands. These glands, situated on top of the kidneys, release hormones that initiate express delivery of energy-giving glucose to cells. This 'express delivery' is much more expensive than ordinary mail, and quickly leads to a deficiency in key nutrients as well as sudden fluctuations in blood sugar and energy levels. This explains why you may experience a dip in energy and concentration a few hours after taking stimulants.

Occasional use of stimulants thus leads to regular use of stimulants and, in due course, as your body's chemistry gets more and more exhausted, you need even more of the stimulant to get the same effect. By now you're a coffee connoisseur, can't function without that cup of tea, or you are addicted to chocolate or cigarettes.

But your body only has a finite capacity to detoxify undesirable substances. Excessive intake of sugar and stimulants,

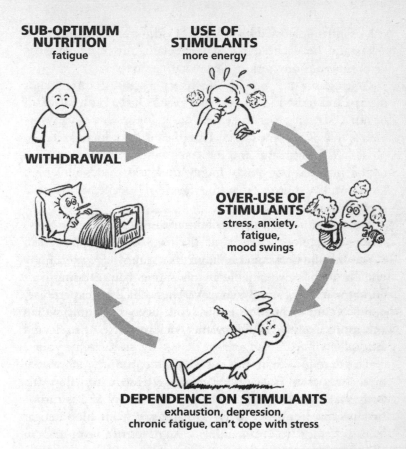

SUB-OPTIMUM NUTRITION
fatigue

USE OF STIMULANTS
more energy

WITHDRAWAL

OVER-USE OF STIMULANTS
stress, anxiety, fatigue, mood swings

DEPENDENCE ON STIMULANTS
exhaustion, depression, chronic fatigue, can't cope with stress

Figure 1 – The vicious circle of stress and fatigue

coupled with sub-optimum nutrition, starts to overload its detoxification potential. And, once you've exceeded this adaptive capacity, your ability to cope with the otherwise normal stresses of modern living becomes compromised.

This can lead to chronic fatigue, allergies, chemical sensitivity, low tolerance of alcohol and smoke, depression, mood swings and feeling out of control. The body is now, effectively, in a state of red alert, and with that comes increased risk of inflammatory diseases such as asthma and eczema, joint aches and headaches. If left unchecked, this can mark the beginning of more serious degenerative diseases.

Getting on the road to recovery requires some major dietary and lifestyle changes. As a result of the body's lack of health reserve, it becomes necessary, for a while, to completely clean up your act. This means avoiding, as far as possible, all stimulants and toxic substances, and focusing on taking into the body only highly nutritious foods plus high levels of key nutrients in the form of specific nutritional supplements.

Once you've built up a good health reserve it isn't necessary to be quite so 'saintly' all the time. A strong body can cope with the occasional indulgence. At this stage your body will let you know quickly if something you're doing isn't good for it. Now, with extra awareness based on experience, you'll be less inclined to ignore your body's warning signals and more likely to avoid another vicious circle of stress and fatigue.

To get to grips with this cycle and find out how to avoid it or recover from it, we need to delve deeper into how the body makes and maintains energy. Its primary fuel is carbohydrate (made up of sugar), so balancing your blood sugar level is critical to maintaining a high energy level and an ability to cope with stress.

PART 1

GENERATING ENERGY

CHAPTER 3

....

BEATING THE SUGAR BLUES

We are all solar-powered – because the energy in food comes from the sun. Plants use the sun's energy to combine water from the soil and carbon dioxide from the air to make carbohydrate; we then eat the plants, break the carbohydrate down into glucose, and release the sun's energy contained within it.

Almost all your energy is derived from glucose – sugar. This is the main 'fuel' of the body and what you eat determines the quality, quantity and availability of glucose to all your body's cells, including the brain. Consequently, maintaining an even blood sugar level is vital in order to ensure good energy levels, mood and overall health. And a key way to control your blood sugar level is by watching what you eat, especially the type of carbohydrate.

All carbohydrates are broken down into sugar which is released into the bloodstream to provide the entire body with fuel. The speed at which this happens affects our energy, mood, weight, ability to deal with stress and our long-term health. Some carbohydrates are 'fast-releasing' (which means they raise blood sugar quickly), while others are 'slow-releasing'. The fast-releasing foods are like rocket fuel. They give a quick burst of energy followed by a rapid burn-out. The slow-releasing foods are more sustaining, giving a consistent energy level. Eating slow-releasing carbohydrates is a vital part of the energy equation.

What makes a food slow- or fast-releasing depends on many factors. Foods contain different kinds of sugars. Most fruits, for example, are rich in slow-releasing fructose, whereas most sweets are rich in fast-releasing sucrose or glucose. The carbohydrates in some foods are complex in structure and take a long time to be digested and broken down into simple sugars. This is true of whole grains such as wholewheat pasta. Some foods contain other ingredients such as fats and fibre that affect the speed at which their carbohydrate content becomes available.

THE GI FACTOR

The rate at which a food releases glucose, or sugar, into your bloodstream can be measured on a scale called the glycaemic index.[1]

When blood sugar levels rise, the body responds by secreting insulin; this hormone sends the sugar into cells or stores it as fat. Glucose is released into the blood after eating, and levels then come down as insulin kicks into action. If a food raises the blood sugar level significantly, and for some time, the area under the blood sugar curve (see Figure 2) is large. Conversely, if a food hardly raises blood glucose levels at all, and then only for a short time, the area under the curve is small.

The amount of food tested obviously affects the height of the blood sugar level. The chart below gives the glycaemic index (GI) score of an average serving of common foods, and will give you some very useful pointers. For example, if you start your day with raisins and puffed rice cereal, both of which have a high GI score, you're setting yourself up for a rapid burn-out. On the other hand, if you kick off with oat flakes, sweetened with a chopped apple (both of which are slow-releasing), your energy will last for longer.

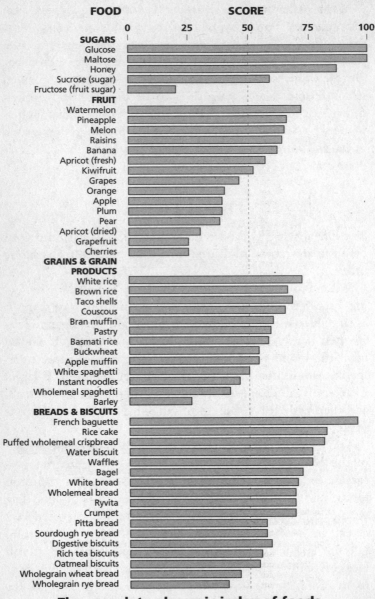

The complete glycemic index of foods

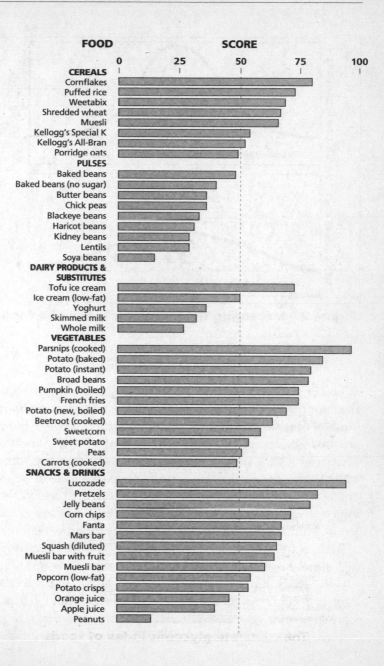

FOOD | SCORE

CEREALS
Cornflakes
Puffed rice
Weetabix
Shredded wheat
Muesli
Kellogg's Special K
Kellogg's All-Bran
Porridge oats
PULSES
Baked beans
Baked beans (no sugar)
Butter beans
Chick peas
Blackeye beans
Haricot beans
Kidney beans
Lentils
Soya beans
DAIRY PRODUCTS & SUBSTITUTES
Tofu ice cream
Ice cream (low-fat)
Yoghurt
Skimmed milk
Whole milk
VEGETABLES
Parsnips (cooked)
Potato (baked)
Potato (instant)
Broad beans
Pumpkin (boiled)
French fries
Potato (new, boiled)
Beetroot (cooked)
Sweetcorn
Sweet potato
Peas
Carrots (cooked)
SNACKS & DRINKS
Lucozade
Pretzels
Jelly beans
Corn chips
Fanta
Mars bar
Squash (diluted)
Muesli bar with fruit
Muesli bar
Popcorn (low-fat)
Potato crisps
Orange juice
Apple juice
Peanuts

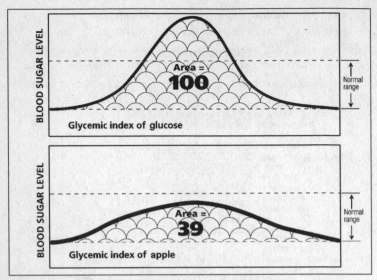

Figure 2 – Measuring the glycaemic index of a food

FOOD COMBINING

Whether a food is fast- or slow-releasing depends on more than just the type of sugar it contains.[2] The presence of certain kinds of fibre slows down the release of sugars, so whole foods are much better for you than refined foods. This means it is better to eat brown rice or wholewheat pasta than the white stuff. It also means that fresh fruit, which contains fibre, is better than fruit juices. The presence of protein in a food also lowers its glycaemic index. That's one reason why beans and lentils, both high in protein and fibre, have such a low GI score.

Thanks to Barry Sears, author of *Enter the Zone*, we now know that combining protein-rich foods with slow-releasing carbohydrates further helps to control blood sugar levels. Protein foods tend to trigger a small, even insulin release. Carbohydrates, especially fast-releasing ones, trigger a large insulin release. Eating fat makes little difference to the insulin response. This advice may go against the grain for people familiar with the food-combining principles of Dr Hay, who advocated not combining protein-rich foods with starches. However, such a diet may be very helpful for people with digestive difficulties, but not in controlling blood sugar levels.

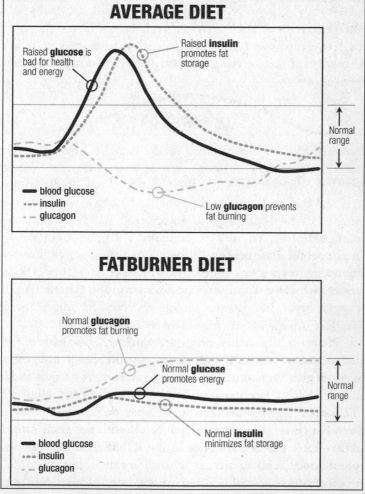

Figure 3 – Blood sugar balance

Generally, foods with a GI score below 50 are very beneficial, while those with a score above 70 should be avoided or
mixed with a low-scoring food. Those with a score between
50 and 70 should be eaten infrequently and only with a low-
scoring food. For example, bananas are quite high, with a
score of 62. Oat flakes and skimmed milk are low, with scores
of 49 and 32 respectively. Having a bowl of oat flakes with
skimmed milk and half a banana for breakfast would therefore
help to keep your blood sugar level on an even keel, while
eating cornflakes (scoring 80) with raisins (scoring 64) would
be bad news.

THE BEST GRAINS

Some grains are better than others because of the type of
carbohydrate they contain. Wheat and corn are high in
amylopectin, which makes them fast-releasing, while barley,
rye and quinoa (a grain which cooks like rice) are higher in
amylose, which makes them slower-releasing. Most rice has a
high GI score because it contains a large proportion of
amylopectin. Basmati rice, however, has more amylose and is
therefore slower-releasing. Brown basmati is best. (One
reason why lentils and soya are so low on the GI scale is that
they contain a substance which prevents the digestion of
amylose, therefore slowing down its release further.)

The way a food is processed makes a difference too.
When wheat is turned into pasta the GI score is low, especially if it is wholemeal. When wheat flour is used to make
bread, cakes, biscuits or pastry, the GI score goes up.
Therefore wholewheat pasta is good, while refined white
bread is bad. The best bread is whole rye grain bread.
There's a world of difference in the GI effect of this and that
of a French baguette.

Of the grains, oats are among the best. While the GI of
wheat varies depending on what's done to it, oats are the

same in any shape or form. Whole oat flakes, rolled oats, or
oatmeal (as used in oatcakes) all have a low glycaemic effect.[3]

THE BEST FRUIT AND VEG

Although most fruits contain fruit sugar, fructose, which is slow-
releasing because it first has to be converted to glucose, some
fruits – such as grapes, pineapples, watermelon and bananas –
also contain varying amounts of fast-releasing glucose. A banana
may be fine when you've just climbed a mountain and need
instant glucose, but it's certainly not the best daily snack. Half
a banana with oats is OK, but oats with chopped apple or pear
is better in terms of keeping your blood sugar level even.

Many 'sugar-free' foods use grape juice concentrate as a
sweetener. This is akin to using glucose. Some use apple juice
concentrate which, being high in fructose, is much better.

Almost all vegetables have a negligible effect on blood
sugar levels. Vegetables that are worth cutting back on are
potatoes, parsnips and swedes which are generally fast-
releasing (boiled new potatoes are slower). Although potato
crisps may have a lower score, this is due to the high fat
content; fat very much slows down the release of glucose
from a food. The same is true of peanuts.

HOW DOES YOUR BODY STORE ENERGY?

If the only way your body could get glucose was directly from
food you'd be dead in two days if you stopped eating. When
you run out of glucose the body breaks down glycogen
(stored in the liver and in muscles) into glucose. When the
glycogen stores are used up, the body burns fat. When the fat
stores are used up, the body burns lean tissue.

Conversely, if your blood glucose level is fine and your
glycogen stores are full, the body stores the fat you eat as fat.
If you eat carbohydrate your body digests this down to

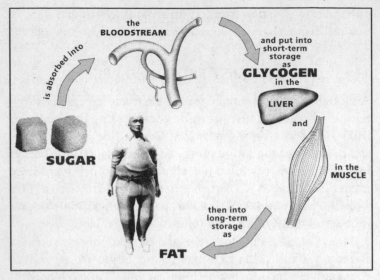

Figure 4 – How the body stores energy as fat

glucose. If your blood glucose level is fine, the liver soaks up this glucose like a sponge and converts it to glycogen. If your glycogen stores are full, it's converted to fat. So, your ability to maintain an even blood sugar level depends not only on what you eat, but also on how efficient your body is at keeping everything in balance by putting excess glucose into storage and, at times of shortage, raiding your energy reserves.

Since every single cell in your body runs on glucose, when there's a shortage not only does your body get tired, so does your mind. You get forgetful, lose concentration and can't think straight. You may also get depressed, irritable and feel unable to cope. These kinds of symptoms are everyday occurrences for many people, who, for one reason or another, lose their ability to keep their blood sugar level even and become over-sensitive to the highs and lows of blood sugar. This is technically called dysglycaemia, or sugar sensitivity, and it is thought to affect about one in four people.

ARE YOU SUGAR SENSITIVE?

How can you find out if you are sugar-sensitive and whether you could benefit from eating the GI way? Nutritionists can run blood tests to find out how you respond; your symptoms and your relationship with sugar are, however, a pretty good guide.

Test Your Sugar Sensitivity

Answer the questions below, ticking those that you answer 'yes' to.

☐ Are you rarely wide awake within 20 minutes of rising?

☐ Do you need tea, coffee, a cigarette or something to get you going in the morning?

☐ Do you really like sweet foods?

☐ Do you crave bread, cereal, popcorn or pasta?

☐ Do you feel like you 'need' an alcoholic drink on most days?

☐ Are you overweight and unable to shift the extra pounds?

☐ Do you often have energy slumps during the day or after meals?

☐ Do you often have mood swings or difficulty concentrating?

☐ Do you get dizzy or irritable if you go six hours without food?

☐ Do you often find you over-react to stress?

☐ Do you frequently get irritable, angry or aggressive unexpectedly?

☐ Do you have less energy now than you used to?

☐ Do you ever lie about how much sweet food you have eaten?

☐ Do you ever keep a supply of sweet food close at hand?

☐ Do you feel you could never give up bread?

If you answer 'yes' to eight or more questions there's a very good chance that you are sugar-sensitive – in other words, struggling to keep your blood sugar level even. Eating the GI way could help you control your blood sugar and energy levels.

In summary, to avoid the dips in energy and mood that come with fluctuating blood sugar levels:

- Avoid sugary foods and drinks.

- Eat foods with a low GI score.

- Combine high-GI-scoring foods with high-protein foods.

The next three chapters deal with stimulants and what happens within cells once glucose arrives.

CHAPTER 4

TURNING FOOD INTO ENERGY

What you experience as energy, whether mental or physical, is the end result of a series of chemical reactions that takes place in every cell in your body. The process that turns food into energy is called catabolism. In a carefully controlled sequence of chemical reactions, food is broken down into its component parts, and these are combusted with oxygen, to make a unit of cellular energy called ATP, which in turn makes muscles work, nerve signals fire and brain cells function. This magical process happens inside every single cell and the only waste products are water and carbon dioxide. But, first of all, the fuel has to be refined.

Although we can make energy from protein, fat and carbohydrate, carbohydrate-rich foods are the best kind of fuel. This is because when fat and protein are used to make energy there is a build-up of toxic substances in the body. Carbohydrates are the only 'smokeless' fuel. Our cells need the simplest unit of carbohydrate, glucose, as fuel. So the first job of the body is to turn all forms of carbohydrate into glucose. This is the end goal of digestion. By eating foods with a low GI score and eating regularly throughout the day, you are giving your cells an even supply of energy-giving glucose.

TURNING GLUCOSE INTO ENERGY

Within each of our thirty trillion or so cells there are tiny energy factories called mitochondria. These are the energy factories of any cell, whether it be a muscle, immune or brain cell. While the cell's instructions, encoded in DNA, come from both parents, the instructions or DNA within these mitochondria come only from the mother. Whether you like it or not, you are more like your mother than your father, and you specifically inherit the same strengths and weaknesses in the energy-producing department.

It is now widely agreed that mitochondria are related to bacteria in the way they work; it is highly likely that early single-celled organisms got infected with bacteria and, in time, the two learnt to live together to mutual advantage, with the bacteria providing the energy for the cell. This allowed the development of more complex cells, of which we are made. Knowing this, you can see why anti-bacterial drugs, such as antibiotics, could have harmful effects on your ability to produce energy, as they may have an effect on the bacteria-like mitochondria.

Many diseases can be traced back to problems with the body's ability to process food for energy within these mitochondria. On the other hand, if you have super-healthy mitochondria, firing on all cylinders, nothing can stop you. So let's examine a little more closely what mitochondria do and how to get them tuned up.

The mitochondria turn glucose into another chemical, pyruvic acid. In this process a small amount of energy is released, which can be used by the cell to carry out its work. But if this step occurs without sufficient oxygen being present, a by-product called lactic acid builds up. That's why the first time you do strenuous exercise, using muscles you didn't even know you had, the next day your muscles ache. This is, in part, because you've made them work too hard without

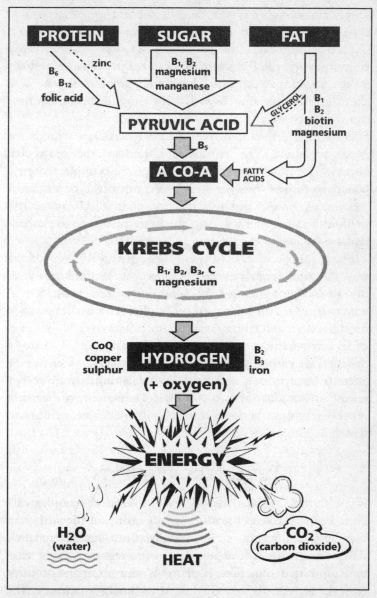

Figure 5 – How mitochondria turn food into energy

supplying enough oxygen, causing a build-up of lactic acid crystals. This is called anaerobic exercise (meaning 'without oxygen'). However, the more you exercise, and develop larger muscles, the less strain you put on the muscles and the more oxygen they can use. This is what aerobic exercise is all about – providing muscle cells with enough oxygen so they can work properly.

Pyruvic acid then gets turned into acetyl-coenzyme A, or AcoA for short. This substance is perhaps the most vital because if you're starved of glucose (for example, when a marathon runner 'hits the wall'), you can break down fat or protein to AcoA, and use this for energy. However this method is rather inefficient so the body prefers to use carbohydrate for fuel.

From this point on, oxygen is needed every step of the way. AcoA undergoes a series of chemical reactions known as the Krebs cycle (named after its discoverer, Ernst Krebs) which separates off hydrogen molecules. The hydrogen then meets oxygen and energy is released. In fact over 90 per cent of all our energy is derived from this final stage. The waste products are carbon dioxide (which we exhale), water (which goes to form urine), and heat. About a third of all energy released from glucose is lost as heat. That's why you get hot when exercising, because muscle cells make lots of energy, which in turn creates heat.

THE ENERGY NUTRIENTS

If you're thinking that all you need to do is eat complex carbohydrates and keep breathing that's only half the story. All these chemical reactions are carefully controlled by enzymes, which are themselves dependent on no less than eight vitamins and five minerals. If there is any shortage of these critical catalysts the output of your energy factories, the mitochondria, is reduced. The result is inefficient energy production, a loss of stamina, highs and lows – or even just lows.

In a survey by the Institute for Optimum Nutrition (ION), 58 per cent of people complained of frequently feeling tired. The researchers found that by simply improving their diet and supplementing the many key vitamins and minerals needed to turn food into energy, 73 per cent of people experienced a definite improvement in their energy levels. This strongly suggests that, for many, the underlying cause of fatigue is simply a lack of the right nutrients.

VITAMIN VITALITY

The important vitamins are the B complex vitamins, a family of eight different substances, every one essential for making energy. Glucose can't be turned into pyruvic acid without B1 and B3 (niacin). AcoA can't be formed without B1, B2, B3, and, most important of all, B5 (pantothenic acid). The Krebs cycle needs B1, B2 and B3 to do its job properly. Fats and proteins can't be used to make energy without B6, B12, folic acid or biotin.

It used to be thought that as long as you ate a reasonable diet you'd get enough B vitamins. But studies have shown that long-term slight deficiencies gradually result in a depletion of these vitamins in cells, causing early warning signs of deficiency such as poor skin condition, anxiety, depression, irritability, and, most of all, fatigue. Many people's diets fall short on these vital vitamins. The Booker Survey in 1985 showed that only one in ten people ate a diet that provided the Recommended Daily Allowance (RDA) for B6 or folic acid.

In one study at the Institute for Optimum Nutrition we gave volunteers, many of whom already had a 'well balanced diet', extra B vitamins in supplement form, often in doses 20 times that of the RDAs. After six months 79 per cent of participants reported a definite improvement in energy, 61 per cent felt physically fitter, and 60 per cent had noticed an improvement in their mental alertness and memory. The likely reason for this is that the RDA levels are not the same as the optimal levels that we need for high-level health and energy.

Because they are water-soluble, if you take in more B vitamins than you need they are simply excreted in your urine. There are a few, like vitamin B6 and vitamin B3, which could become toxic if you were to consume several grams but who would want to do that? Because of their water-solubility and sensitivity to heat, B vitamins are also easily lost when foods are boiled in water. The best natural sources are therefore fresh fruit, raw vegetables, and wheat-germ. Seeds, nuts and wholegrains contain reasonable amounts, as do meat, fish, eggs and dairy produce. But these levels are reduced when the food is cooked or stored for a long time.

The final stage before energy can be derived by reacting hydrogen with oxygen is also dependent on a special co-enzyme, co-enzyme Q (Co-Q). A vital link in the chain, Co-Q provides the spark, fuelled by oxygen, which keeps your energy furnace burning.

CO-ENZYME Q

The discovery that Co-Q is present in foods, that levels decline with age, and that cellular levels rise when supplements are taken, has led many nutritionists to suspect that Co-Q may be the missing link in the energy equation. Technically, Co-Q cannot be classified as a vitamin since it can be made by the body (even if it isn't made in large enough amounts for optimum health and energy). It is therefore a semi-essential nutrient.

Co-Q 'magically' improves the cell's ability to use oxygen.

In the final and most significant part of catabolism, when hydrogen is released during the Krebs cycle to react with oxygen, the actual reaction occurs at an atomic level. The components of these elements, called electrons, are passed from one atom to the next, in what is called the electron transfer pathway. These electrons, which are tiny charged particles, are highly reactive and need to be very carefully handled. They are like nuclear fuel – a very potent but very dangerous energy source.

So dangerous are these spare electrons that they are thought to initiate the process that makes some cells become cancerous, and damages cells within artery walls, heralding the beginning of heart disease. The damage caused to healthy cells by these spare electrons is a large part of what constitutes ageing. The more damaged cells we have, the older we are biochemically. Compounds that contain spare electrons are called free radicals. They are created during normal energy catabolism, but also when we smoke, eat fried food, breathe in pollution, and when we are exposed to radiation from the sun. Co-Q has two key roles to play in handling these volatile electrons. It controls the flow of oxygen, making the production of energy most efficient, and prevents damage caused by these free radicals.

CO-Q IS SAFE AND EFFECTIVE

I am not aware of any studies that have reported toxicity of Co-Q, even at extremely high doses taken over many years. There is no reason to assume that continued supplementation with Co-Q, as is advised for many vitamins, should have anything but extremely positive results.

Co-Q is in many foods but not always in a form that we can make use of directly. There are many different types of Co-Q (from Co-Q1 to Co-Q10). Yeast, for example, contains Co-Q6 and Co-Q7. Only Co-Q10 is found in human tissues. It is this form of Co-Q that is effective in the ways described in this book and only this form should be supplemented. However, we can utilise 'lower' forms of Co-Q and convert them into Co-Q10. This conversion process, which occurs in the liver, allows us to make use of the Co-Q found in almost all foods.

But some people, especially the elderly find it difficult or impossible to convert lower forms of Co-Q into the active Co-Q10. We do not know exactly why, or to what extent their ability to do this is impaired. But for these people Co-Q10 is effectively an essential nutrient; in other words, their bodies need to be given a supply of it. This is probably why deficiency in Co-Q occurs.

Some foods contain relatively more Co-Q10, and these foods are probably our best dietary sources of Co-Q. These include all meat and fish (especially sardines), eggs, spinach, broccoli, alfalfa, potato, soya beans and soya oil, wheat (especially wheatgerm), rice bran, buckwheat, millet, and most beans, nuts and seeds.

Best Food Sources of Co-enzyme Q10

(milligrams per gram)

Food	Amount	Food	Amount
Meat		**Beans**	
Beef	.031	Green beans	.0058
Pork	.024–.041	Soya beans	.0029
Chicken	.021	Aduki beans	.0022
Fish		**Nuts and Seeds**	
Sardine	.064	Peanuts	.027
Mackerel	.043	Sesame seeds	.023
Flat fish	.005	Walnuts	.019

Grains		Vegetables	
Rice bran	.0054	Spinach	.010
Rice	–	Broccoli	.008
Wheatgerm	.0035	Peppers	.003
Wheatflour	–	Carrots	.002
Millet	.0015	**Oils**	
Buckwheat	.0013	Soya oil	.092

Today, many supplement companies offer Co-Q10 products. The best dosage is probably between 10 and 90mg a day and it is best absorbed in an oil-soluble form.

ELEMENTAL ENERGY

The minerals iron, calcium, magnesium, chromium and zinc are also vital for making energy. Calcium and magnesium are perhaps the most important because all muscle cells need an adequate supply of these to be able to contract and relax. A shortage of magnesium (very common in people who don't eat much fruit or vegetables) often results in cramps, as muscles are unable to relax.

Magnesium is needed by 75 per cent of the enzymes in your body[4] – and it is vital for carbohydrate metabolism. It is also essential for nerve cells to send their messages. Symptoms of deficiency include muscle tremors, muscle weakness, insomnia, nervousness, hyperactivity, depression, confusion, irregular heartbeat, constipation and lack of appetite. Most of these are connected with impaired muscle or nerve function.

We need zinc, together with vitamin B6, to make the enzymes that digest food.[5] They are also essential in the production of the hormone insulin, which helps to control blood sugar levels. A lack of zinc also disturbs our appetite control mechanism and reduces our senses of taste or smell, often leading to over-consumption of meat, cheese and other strong-tasting foods.

The older you are, the less likely you are to be taking in enough chromium,[6] an essential mineral that helps stabilise blood sugar levels. The average daily intake is below 50mcg, whereas the optimal intake, certainly for those with blood sugar problems, is around 200mcg. Chromium is found in wholefoods and is therefore higher in wholewheat flour, bread and pasta than in refined products; it is also present in beans, nuts and seeds. Asparagus and mushrooms are especially rich in chromium. Since it works with insulin to help stabilise your blood sugar level, the more uneven your blood sugar level the more chromium you use up. Hence, a sugar and stimulant addict, eating refined foods, is most at risk of deficiency. Flour has 98 per cent of its chromium removed in the refining process – another reason to stay away from refined foods.

Whether or not you can achieve an optimal intake of chromium from diet alone is debatable. It is therefore wise to take supplements as well as eating wholefoods. The best forms of chromium are either picolinate or polynicotinate. Chromium polynicotinate is chromium bound with niacin (vitamin B3). Chromium is part of a special molecule produced by the liver, called Glucose Tolerance Factor, whose structure includes chromium, niacin and the amino acids cystine, glycine and glutamic acid.

SUPPLEMENTS FOR ENERGY

To maintain a consistently high energy level, you need to optimise your intake of all the nutrients involved in turning food into energy, as well as making sure you eat the right kinds of food. One of the easiest ways to guarantee such optimal levels is to take nutritional supplements. These are the daily amounts to aim for (see Chapter 19 to work out your ideal supplement programme):

B1 (thiamine)	25–100mg
B2 (riboflavin)	25–100mg
B3 (niacin)	50–150mg
B5 (pantothenic acid)	50–200mg
B6 (pyridoxine)	50–100mg
B12 (cyanocobalamin)	10–100mcg
Folic acid	100–400mcg
Biotin	50–150mcg
Co-enzyme Q10	10–90mg
Vitamin C	1000–3000mg
Calcium	150–500mg
Magnesium	100–3000mg
Iron	5–15mg
Zinc	10–20mg
Chromium	100–300mcg

These levels can be achieved by taking a high-strength multi-vitamin and multimineral, plus an additional 1000mg vitamin C and 100–200mcg chromium, depending on how much is in your multimineral.

In summary, to maintain a high energy level, you need to:

- Eat foods rich in B vitamins (e.g. wheatgerm, fish, green vegetables, wholegrains, mushrooms and eggs).

- Eat foods rich in vitamin C (e.g. peppers, watercress, cabbage, broccoli, cauliflower, strawberries, lemons, kiwi fruit, oranges and tomatoes).

- Eat foods rich in Co-Q (e.g. sardines, mackerel, sesame seeds, peanuts, walnuts and pork).

- Eat foods rich in magnesium (e.g. wheatgerm, almonds, cashew nuts, buckwheat and green vegetables), calcium (e.g. cheese, almonds, green vegetables, seeds and prunes), zinc (e.g. oysters, lamb, nuts, fish, egg yolk, wholegrains and almonds), and iron (e.g. pumpkin seeds, almonds, cashew nuts, raisins and pork).

■ Take a high-strength multivitamin and multimineral, plus extra vitamin C (1000 mg) and chromium (200 mcg).

CHAPTER 5

....

ARE YOU ADDICTED TO STRESS AND STIMULANTS?

Whatever thoughts you have about stress, the reality is that body chemistry fundamentally changes every time a person reacts to it. Stress starts in the mind. We perceive a situation as requiring our immediate attention – a young child getting too close to the road, a car getting too close to us, an impossible deadline, a hostile reaction from someone, having to call the bank manager to increase your overdraft facility. Rapid signals stimulate the adrenal glands (situated on top of your kidneys, in the small of your back) to produce adrenalin. Within seconds your heart is pounding, your breathing changes, stores of glucose are released into your blood, your muscles tense, your eyes dilate, your blood thickens.

What, you might ask, has all this got to do with calling your bank manager? The answer is: very little. But, before the days of overdraft facilities, most stressful situations required a physical response. That's what adrenalin does. It gets you ready to 'fight or take flight'. The average adrenalin rush experienced by a commuter stuck in a traffic jam is enough to keep them running for a mile. That's how much glucose is released, mainly by breaking down glycogen held in muscles and the liver.

To get the fuel into the body cells, the pancreas releases two hormones, insulin and glucagon. Insulin helps carry the fuel out of the blood; glucagon tops up the blood sugar if the level gets too low. Another substance, released from the liver,

Glucose Tolerance Factor, potentiates the effect of insulin. All this is happening as a result of a stressful thought.

Where, you might wonder, does all this extra energy and increased alertness come from? The answer is that it is diverted from the body's normal repair and maintenance jobs such as digesting, cleansing and rejuvenating. So, every moment you spend under stress, the ageing process of your body speeds up. It's stressful even thinking about it! But the effects of prolonged stress are even more insidious. Imagine your pituitary and adrenal glands, pancreas and liver perpetually pumping out hormones to control blood sugar that you don't even need, day in, day out. Like a car driven too fast, your body soon goes out of balance and parts start to wear out.

THE BLOOD SUGAR BLUES

As a consequence your energy level drops, you lose concentration, get confused, suffer from bouts of 'brain fag', fall asleep after meals, get irritable, freak out, can't sleep, can't wake up, sweat too much, get headaches . . . does this sound familiar? In an attempt to regain control, most people turn to stimulants. Legal stimulants include coffee (containing theobromine, theophylline and caffeine), tea (containing caffeine), sweet fizzy drinks including Lucozade (containing caffeine), chocolate (containing theophylline), cigarettes (containing nicotine), and psychological 'stimulants', including demanding jobs, dangerous pastimes, horror movies, thrillers, emotional traumas – something to put you 'on the edge'. Illegal stimulants include amphetamines and 'uppers', cocaine, crack and crime. Living on stimulants, it naturally becomes increasingly difficult to relax. Many people counter this by learning to use relaxants such as alcohol, sleeping pills, tranquillisers, cannabis and so on. While the immediate effect of these substances are as a relaxant, the long-term effect is often to generate anxiety.

ADDICTED TO STRESS

Of course, you can't live like this forever, so most people burn out and have to head for the beach to recover. And while they wait in the airport, what better way to relax than by reading a novel? The back cover says 'murder, mystery, greed, lust, gripping suspense'. Sounds good. After two tense hours of fictional murder, mystery and intrigue on the beach it's time for some real excitement – perhaps windsurfing or waterskiing? What is it we're looking for?

In an interview with Evel Knievel in the cockpit of his 'rocket bike' an interviewer asked 'Why do you do it?' Evel replied, 'There is a moment, when I'm flying through the air, of absolute peace.' He closed the hatch, pressed the button and seconds later the rocket slammed into the side of the Grand Canyon. I first heard this story in the introduction to a meditation course. The speaker concluded by saying, 'There must be an easier way than this.' The point is that many people become physiologically addicted to the very potent cocktail of chemical 'uppers' and 'downers' triggered by stress.

Instead of using these hormones as a back-up, a super-charge only to be called on in times of emergency, many people live on adrenalin and other stress hormones such as cortisol all the time, relying on coffee, tea, cigarettes or sugar. After a while, it's only the adrenalin that keeps them going. If they quit the stimulants or take some time off, they collapse in a heap – depressed and exhausted. This means they've become addicted to stress and/or stimulants.

ARE YOU ADDICTED TO STIMULANTS?

Imagine a day with no coffee, tea, sugar, chocolate, cigarettes or alcohol. If you shudder at the very thought it's quite possible that you have some level of addiction to stimulants. This can range from a mild addiction that you can live with quite happily to a major addiction that is running your life. However, whatever your level of addiction, the net consequence is less energy rather than more.

One of our clients, Bobbie, is a case in point. She was already eating a healthy diet and took a sensible daily programme of vitamin and mineral supplements. She had only two problems (a lack of energy in the morning and occasional headaches) and one vice: three cups of coffee a day. After some persuasion she agreed to stop coffee for one month. To her surprise, up went her energy level and the headaches stopped.

In order to assess your current relationship with stimulants it is very helpful to be honest about your actual intake. Keep a daily diary for just three days. Note down how much and when you consume: coffee, tea, chocolate, sugar (or something sweet), cigarettes or alcohol.

Also, think about your relationship with these substances. Do you, for example, ever buy sweets and hide the wrappers so other people won't know? Do you always order a dessert at restaurants, and take a mint or two on the way out? How much do you look forward to that cup of coffee in the morning or in your lunch break? How important is that drink after work? How secretive are you about the amount you smoke? Have you become a coffee connoisseur, side-stepping the issue of addiction by focusing on your hobby of sampling yet another type of freshly ground coffee? This kind of relationship with stimulants, often cloaked in the attitude that these are just the normal pleasures of life, is indicative of an underlying chemical imbalance that depletes your energy and peace of mind.

You don't need stimulants

Stimulants are energy's greatest enemy. Even though stimulants can create energy in the short term, the long-term effect is always bad. The same is true of stress. So the first step to beating stress and fatigue is to cut out, or cut down on stimulants. This includes coffee, tea, chocolate, sugar and refined foods, cigarettes, cola drinks and alcohol.

Stop your intake of these stimulants for one month and notice what happens. The more damage stimulants are doing to you, the greater the withdrawal effect. (Fortunately, by eating slow-releasing carbohydrates and taking energy nutrients as supplements you can minimise the withdrawal symptoms which usually last no more than four days.)

Then start again and notice what happens when you have your first cup of tea, coffee, or hit of sugar or chocolate. You'll experience what Hans Selye (who described the

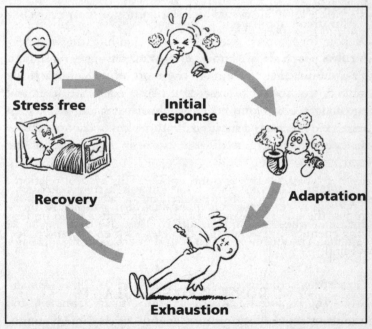

Figure 6 – The general adaptation syndrome

General Adaptation Syndrome in Figure 6) called the 'initial response' – in other words a true response to these powerful chemicals: a pounding head, hyperactive mind, fast heartbeat, insomnia, followed by extreme drowsiness. Keep taking the stimulants and you will adapt – that's phase 2. Keep doing this long enough and eventually you will hit exhaustion – phase 3. This happens to everybody. The only variable is how long it takes a person to get to the 'exhaustion' phase.

Yet recovery is not only possible, it's usually rapid. Most people feel substantially more energetic and able to cope with stress within 30 days of quitting stimulants, with nutritional support.

WHAT'S REALLY IN STIMULANTS?

It's worth knowing what the most common stimulants contain and how they affect your body.

Alcohol   is made by the action of yeast on sugar. As such, it has a similar effect to sugar. In the short term alcohol actually inhibits the release of reserve glucose from the liver and encourages low blood sugar levels, causing an increase in appetite. Diseases associated with excess alcohol intake include diabetes, heart disease, cirrhosis and cancer of the liver.

Chocolate   contains cocoa as its major 'active' ingredient. Cocoa provides significant quantities of the stimulant theobromine, whose action is similar to, though not as strong as, caffeine. Theobromine is also found in cocoa drinks, like hot chocolate.

Cigarettes   contain nicotine, as well as 16 other cancer-producing chemicals. Nicotine is the primary stimulant and has a substantial effect even in small doses. In large amounts, nicotine acts as a sedative. It is more addictive than heroin.

People breaking the habit often experience low blood sugar problems.

Coffee   contains theobromine, theophylline and caffeine, all of which are stimulants. Caffeine is the major stimulant, but decaffeinated coffee still contains the other two. Theophylline disturbs normal sleep patterns. Coffee consumption is associated with greater risk of cancer of the pancreas and, during pregnancy, increased incidence of birth defects.

Fizzy drinks   can contain a quarter of the caffeine found in a weak cup of coffee. They usually contain sugar and colourings which also act as stimulants.

Medications   for the relief of headaches may contain caffeine. Other caffeine tablets are available as stimulants. The most common are Pro Plus and the herb Guarana.

Tea   contains caffeine, theobromine, theophylline and tannin. It is a stimulant and a diuretic with similar, though lesser effects to coffee. A strong cup of tea can provide as much caffeine as a weak cup of coffee. Tannin interferes with the absorption of minerals. Tea drinkers have an increased risk of stomach ulcers.

REDUCING STIMULANTS WITHOUT SUFFERING

Of course cutting all these stimulants out completely would be just about impossible for many people, and certainly stressful! The first step is to find out which are most important for you. Start by looking at your habits. Which of these stimulants, if any, do you have in one form or another several times a day? Which do you use as a pick-me-up, perhaps to get you out of bed in the morning or when your energy is flagging during the day? Which would you find the hardest to cut out completely for one month? When was the last time you went for one month without each of these stimulants?

Although you may intend to stop them for ever, in reality it is a lot easier to take one step at a time. So start by picking one stimulant (other than cigarettes) which you use frequently. Could you realistically cut it out for one month only? If not, what could you reduce your intake to? Write this down and stick to it. Set yourself similar targets for no more than three stimulants. Sometimes they overlap. For example, if you use coffee, sugar and chocolate, but can't stand coffee without sugar, then cutting out sugar automatically means no chocolate and no coffee.

Here are some tips to help you get started.

Sugar   is an acquired taste. Although we are born with a liking for sweet things, research has shown that only those who are regularly fed sweets and sweet foods like high levels of sweetness. So, as you gradually cut down the level of sweetness in *all* the food you eat, you will soon get accustomed to this. This means having less sugar in hot drinks, less in food, less dried fruit, and drinking more diluted fruit juice. When you want something sweet have fruit. Sweeten cereals and desserts with fruit, and if you're really desperate have a Fruitus cereal bar, or Rebar fruit and veg bar (available from any healthfood shop) instead of chocolate or sweets.

Don't replace sugar with sugar substitutes. These may not raise your blood sugar levels, but neither do they allow you to change your habits. It takes about a month to acquire a preference for less sweet foods. Let your tastebuds be the judge of how sweet a food is – but do check the labels for all those disguised forms of sugar.

Coffee   is strongly addictive. It takes, on average, four days to break the habit. During these days you may experience headaches and grogginess. These are a strong reminder of how bad coffee really is for you. Decaffeinated coffee is only slightly better. The most popular coffee alternatives are Caro, Dandex, Barleycup and Symington's Dandelion coffee.

When you have been off coffee for a month you may decide the occasional cup would be nice. Have this as a treat, perhaps when you eat out, not as a pick-me-up.

Tea is not as bad for you as coffee, unless you're the sort of person that likes your tea well stewed. Start by decreasing the strength of your tea, perhaps using a smaller cup or teapot. Tea has such a strong flavour that you can literally dip in a tea bag for seconds and still have a strong-tasting drink. Use Luaka tea, which is a good-quality Ceylon tea that is naturally low in tannin and caffeine. The most popular alternatives are herb teas such as Celestial Seasonings (Red Zinger and Mandarin Orange are my favourites) or Yogi Teas. Red Bush (or Rooibos) tea is good with milk and has a taste closer to 'normal' tea.

Chocolate contains both sugar and chocolate. Start by having chocolate-free snacks. Then switch to chocolate- and sugar-free snacks. Eventually you can avoid even these, keeping them strictly for emergencies and eating fresh fruit instead if you feel you need something sweet.

Alcohol is an easy habit to acquire because of its key role in social interaction. Start by limiting the times when you have alcohol. For example, don't drink at lunchtime; you'll certainly work better in the afternoon. Then limit what you drink. For example, stick to wine, and avoid beer or spirits. Limit how much you drink by setting yourself a weekly target – for example, seven glasses of wine a week. This allows you to have quite a few at that party on Saturday night and compensate by having little throughout the preceding week. Ideally, you should cut it out completely for at least the first two weeks. If you find this hard to do take a close look at your drinking habits, and, if necessary, seek professional help.

Smoking can be one of the hardest habits to kick. But improved nutrition decreases your craving for cigarettes so it's best to leave this one until you've been following the recommendations in this book for at least two months. Once you have done this, follow the guidelines given in the next chapter.

In summary, to break your addiction to stress and stimulants, you need to:

- Identify which stimulants you are addicted to.

- Find which substitutes you like most and avoid or considerably reduce your intake of stimulants until they are no longer a daily requirement.

- Stop smoking, following the guidelines in the next chapter.

- Notice the way you behave when under stress and replace these behaviour patterns with healthier ones (e.g. eating fruit instead of sweets or chocolates).

CHAPTER 6

HOW TO QUIT SMOKING

One of the hardest stimulants to give up is cigarettes. Cigarettes contain nicotine, as well as 16 other cancer-producing chemicals. Nicotine, the primary stimulant, is more addictive than heroin and it produces a substantial effect even in small doses. In large amounts, it acts as a sedative. This is the attraction of nicotine: on the one hand it can give you a lift, on the other it can calm you down. Before a meal it can stop you feeling hungry and after a meal it can stop you feeling drowsy.

All these effects are due to nicotine's action on adrenal hormones, blood sugar and brain chemicals. If you follow the advice given in Parts 1 and 2 of this book your craving for cigarettes will diminish. This is a direct consequence of stabilising your blood sugar and hormone levels.

Before attempting to give up cigarettes you should follow these diet and supplement guidelines strictly for two months, preferably with the guidance and support of a clinical nutritionist, until you no longer consume any other stimulants (such as tea, coffee and chocolate) or sugar. Instead, eat small, frequent meals containing slow-releasing carbohydrates combined with protein-rich foods.

Breaking the Associated Habits

The average smoker is not only addicted to nicotine, but is also addicted to smoking when tired, hungry or upset, on waking, after a meal, with a drink and so on. Before you actually give up smoking altogether it is best to break these mental associations.

Without attempting to change your smoking habits, keep a diary for a week, writing down every situation in which you smoke, how you feel before and how you feel after smoking. You can copy the opposite page to record your one-week smoking diary.

When the week is up, add up how many cigarettes you have smoked, associated with each situation. Your list might look something like this:

With a hot drink –16
After a meal –14
With alcohol –20
Difficult situation – 4
After sex – 3

Now set yourself fortnightly targets. For the first two weeks smoke as much as you like whenever you like but not when you drink a hot drink. For the next two weeks smoke as much as you like whenever you like but not when you drink a hot drink or within 30 minutes of finishing a meal. Continue like this until, when you smoke, all you do is smoke, without the associated habits.

This will be tremendously helpful for you when you quit. Most people start again because the phone rings with a problem, someone brings in a coffee, offers you a cigarette . . . and before you know it you're smoking.

Day _____			
Time	Situation	Feeling Before	Feeling After
9am	With coffee	Tired	Awake

Figure 7 – Smoking diary

REDUCING YOUR NICOTINE LOAD

Now it's time to reduce your nicotine load gradually. Week by week, switch to a brand that contains less nicotine until what you smoke contains no more than 2mg per cigarette. In addition to the supplements recommended in Chapter 19, supplementing 1000mg vitamin C, 100mcg chromium and 50mg niacin with each meal should help reduce your cravings. You may experience a blushing sensation when first taking niacin. This is harmless and usually occurs 15 to 30 minutes after taking it, for about 15 minutes. The blushing is less likely to occur if you take niacin with a meal and will diminish and, in most cases, stop completely if you take 50mg three times a day.

Increasing the alkaline balance of the body helps reduce cravings: one way to achieve this is by eating a diet that is high in fruit, vegetables and seeds. In addition, consider supplementing calcium (600mg) and magnesium (400mg) daily, as these are alkaline minerals and help to neutralise excess acidity.

Whenever you feel the need for nicotine first eat an apple or pear. This will raise a low blood sugar level, which is often the factor that triggers such a craving.

Regular exercise also helps, so this is a great time to sign up at your local gym, start jogging or learn Psychocalisthenics (see Chapter 13).

Now reduce the number of cigarettes until you are smoking no more than five cigarettes a day, each with a nicotine content of 2mg or less. If you wish, stop smoking and replace with nicotine gum as an intermediate step. Nicotine gum comes in two strengths – 4mg and 2mg.

You want to get down to a maximum of 10mg of nicotine a day before quitting i.e. five pieces of 2mg nicotine gum, or five 2mg nicotine cigarettes.

TIME TO QUIT

It is now time to quit and it is best to give yourself all the support you can get. Make sure your friends and work colleagues know so they can support you, rather than over-reacting if you are not at your best. It's great to have a friend you can talk to whenever you are craving nicotine. They can help strengthen your resolve.

The withdrawal effects from nicotine are a direct result of its action on your blood sugar, adrenal hormone levels and key chemicals in the brain. It is vital to follow a really good nutritional programme during the first month after quitting. Make sure you always have a good breakfast, lunch and dinner and have low GI snacks (see Chapter 3) available during the day whenever your blood sugar levels dip.

You may also find it helpful to take a 5-Hydroxy-Tryptophan (5-HTP) supplement. This is an amino acid that is converted in the body into serotonin, an important brain chemical that controls mood. Nicotine withdrawal tends to reduce serotonin levels, leading to depression and irritability. By supplementing 200mg of 5-HTP (available from health-food stores), you can prevent this happening. It's best to take 5-HTP on an empty stomach or with a piece of fruit, one hour before you go to bed. (Serotonin levels rise at night, promoting a good night's sleep.)

Another useful aid during the first month is licorice, which promotes the action of adrenal hormones. Since nicotine acts as an adrenal stimulant, this additional adrenal support can be helpful during the withdrawal phase. Licorice is either available as a supplement or as a bar. The only bar I'd recommend is Panda licorice, which is sweetened with molasses rather than sugar.

In supplement form, the dose is 1–2g powdered root or 2–4ml fluid extract (1 : 1 strength) three times a day. Check the manufacturer's instructions, as potencies can vary. Licorice should be avoided or used with caution by people with high blood pressure – ask your GP to check your blood pressure and visit a qualified herbalist for expert advice.

DETOXIFYING YOUR BODY

To reduce your craving for cigarettes, you need to boost your body's ability to detoxify and eliminate chemicals, including nicotine. There are five things you can do to speed up this process. These are exercise, sweating, drinking plenty of water and supplementing vitamin C and niacin. Putting all these together adds up to a winning formula for rapid detox-ification.

If you have access to a sauna or steam room at a gym here's what to do:

- Take 1g vitamin C and 100mg niacin.

- Go for a run or do any cardiovascular exercise that raises your pulse rate and stimulates your circulation.

- Once you start blushing as a consequence of the niacin, go into the sauna or steam room. The sauna should never be at a temperature above 80°F.

- Take in 1 litre of water and keep drinking it at regular inter-vals.

Take a sauna for half an hour every day. (This routine is not recommended for those with a history of cardiovascular dis-ease, except under medical supervision. While no danger is anticipated or reported the combination of exercise, niacin and saunas is a substantial stimulation to circulation, and hence cellular detoxification, which is the purpose of this routine.)

CHAPTER 7

....

BALANCING THE STRESS HORMONES

By now you will be starting to realise that what you eat, drink and smoke has a profound effect on how you feel. But how exactly does this work? By what means do these stimulants affect your mood? The answer is hormones. Hormones affect key chemicals in your brain that change your whole perception of life and your environment.

There are two main biochemical reasons why people become addicted to stress and/or stimulants. The first is that they can raise a low blood sugar level, thus temporarily improving energy levels. The second is that they can stimulate the release of adrenal hormones, providing a boost to keep you going through the day. An understanding of how these chemicals of communication work is very helpful in solving the stress syndrome.

THE DANCE OF THE HORMONES

Hormones are chemical messengers. They are special chemicals, produced in special cells (collectively known as endocrine glands, e.g. the adrenal gland or thyroid gland), that are released into the bloodstream to deliver their instructions to targeted body cells.

We've already met a few of them. Insulin helps take sugar out of the blood; glucagon raises a low blood sugar level by calling on sugar reserves stored as glycogen and fat; adrenalin raises blood sugar levels by breaking down glycogen; cortisol, another adrenal hormone, stimulates the liver to make glucose from protein.

And there's one more adrenal hormone which helps maintain energy and stress resistance. That's dehydro-epiandrosterone (DHEA), the cousin of cortisol.

When all these hormones are in balance so are you. Your energy level is good, your mind is sharp, and so-called stress becomes simply another problem to solve. Before explaining how they all link together and how to bring them into balance it's worth knowing how they relate to each other chemically.

Insulin, glucagon and adrenalin are proteins. This means they are made from a particular arrangement of amino acids that come from protein in food. Other nutrients are also used in making their chemical structure. For example, insulin requires zinc and vitamin B6, while adrenalin requires vitamin C and B12, among others.

Cortisol and DHEA are fat-based compounds known as steroid hormones. They are made from cholesterol which the body can synthesise. These two hormones are chemically very similar and have a profound effect on each other. The amount of cortisol and DHEA a person produces shows where they are in the stress cycle (see Figure 8). The sex hormones oestrogen, progesterone and testosterone are also made from cholesterol, which is why excessive stress can lead to hormone-related problems in both men and women.

HOW HORMONES AFFECT YOUR BLOOD SUGAR LEVELS

Just like the pieces in a chess game, each hormone can affect another in a specific way. Here's how it works.

If you eat a meal containing fast-releasing carbohydrates, up goes your blood sugar. Insulin is then released to get the excess glucose out of your blood, into cells as fuel or into storage. If your blood sugar level isn't quite high enough (perhaps because it's on the rebound, or because it's been a while since you last ate), glucagon is released which makes more glucose available. It does this by breaking down short-term reserves of glycogen, held in the liver and in muscles.

If the blood sugar level goes too low this also stimulates the release of adrenal hormones, which perceive this lack of vital fuel as an emergency. The adrenal hormones have one mission in life – your survival. If ever your survival is threatened they leap into action. This will happen if you injure yourself, undergo surgery, are shocked (perhaps by the flash of a speed trap), skip a meal or have a rebound low blood sugar level from eating the wrong kind of food. The body first releases adrenalin, the effects of which only last a short time (up to an hour). Then DHEA and cortisol kick in.

Between them they have many effects, all designed to make sure you've got the fuel to 'fight or take flight'. So, whenever your blood sugar level dips too low, in come the adrenal hormones to get your blood sugar level up again. Most of us are well aware of these dynamics and help the process along by stimulating the release of adrenalin when our blood sugar level is low – for instance, by having a coffee.

The problem is that the extra energy liberated by adrenal stimulation comes at a price. In the long term, it suppresses your immune system, slows down your body's rate of repair and slows down your body's metabolism. In other words, the cost of going into 'stress survival mode' frequently or for long periods is rapid ageing, weight gain and a greater risk of osteoporosis and degenerative disease.

As we learnt in the last chapter we can't keep doing this forever. The body adapts to stress and then finally mal-adapts, going into a state of exhaustion. At this point you can't cope with stress and feel exhausted. Knowing where you are in the cycle is the key to finding the best way out.

THE STRESS CYCLE

Stage 1 – The Initial Response

What we know as stress (for example, meeting a tough deadline) stimulates the pituitary gland in the brain which releases ACTH, a hormone which stimulates the adrenal cortex. As a result your levels of DHEA and cortisol go up. When these are high enough the brain stops producing ACTH. Once the stress is over, your cortisol and DHEA levels return to normal.

Stage 2 – Adaptation

With repeated stress the body becomes tired and less responsive to the effects of cortisol. This calls for more cortisol to be

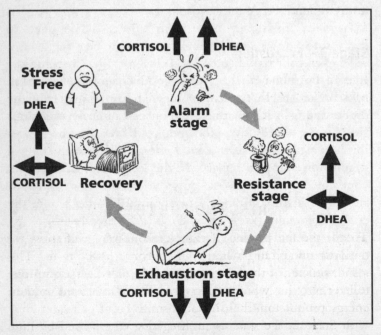

Figure 8 – The stress cycle

produced. Since DHEA can be turned into cortisol, the body makes this extra cortisol at the expense of DHEA. Cortisol levels are therefore raised and DHEA levels fall. As it takes more time for these adrenal hormones to raise blood sugar levels to normal, you feel tired and less able to keep your energy level on an even keel.

In time adaptation turns to mal-adaptation. Your cortisol level keeps going up, while your DHEA level keeps falling since your body can no longer produce adequate levels of both. You start to suffer from chronic fatigue and show signs of poor immunity (because the adrenal hormones shut down your immune system). Now you are becoming more prone to infections and finding them harder to shift. At this stage you are reacting more strongly to stress and finding it hard to return to normal. Being in a permanent state of stress becomes a way of life.

Stage 3 – Exhaustion

Eventually your body can't even produce enough cortisol so both this and DHEA are low. You fall to pieces with even the slightest stress, get irritable, can't concentrate, have no energy and get depressed. You may get headaches, can no longer tolerate alcohol and become prone to inflammatory and degenerative disease.

STRESS AND THE THYROID

To get the full picture of this hormonal game of stress we need to understand where the thyroid gland fits in. This gland, situated at the base of the throat, produces a hormone called thyroxine which effectively tells cells to speed up their energy production, their metabolism.

In Stage 2, the state of prolonged stress, marked by high cortisol levels, your thyroxine levels fall. This is because the adrenal hormone cortisol is directly antagonistic to thyroxine, presumably trying to conserve energy by slowing down metabolism in what it perceives as an emergency situation. As a result thyroxine levels in your blood fall and so does your body temperature.

Thyroid tests measure two things: the level of Thyroid Stimulating Hormone (TSH) and the level of thyroxine. TSH is produced by the pituitary gland in the brain and it tells the thyroid gland to produce more thyroxine. It produces two kinds of thyroxine, one of which is called T4, which is a kind of 'pre-hormone' that gets converted into T3, the active hormone. It's the T3 level that counts.

When cortisol levels are raised under stress, TSH levels fall. So there's less stimulation of the thyroid gland. Also, cortisol stops the inactive T4 turning into the active T3. So low TSH and low T3 are other indicators of prolonged stress.

TEST YOUR STRESS

You can pinpoint exactly where you are in this cycle of stress by measuring your levels of all these hormones. This is best done by analysing saliva hormone levels rather than blood. The reason for this is that, once hormones are released, most get attached to proteins in the blood. Only a small amount of the hormone is 'free', unattached and able to deliver the message. The 'free' hormone level is reflected better in saliva than in blood. The respective levels and the relationship between cortisol and DHEA show where you are in the stress cycle. The Adrenal Stress Index (ASI) test is available through nutrition consultants who are trained to devise the most effective regime to rapidly rebalance your stress hormonal levels – a process that normally takes four to eight weeks.

Your pulse and blood pressure are also directly influenced by your adrenalin levels. When you are unstressed and lying down, which is the state you should be in on rising, your pulse will naturally be lower, as will your blood pressure. The mere act of standing up raises adrenalin and consequently your pulse and blood pressure. If your blood pressure is high and there is no change in your blood pressure from lying down to standing up, or if your pulse rate upon waking is high (80+ beats a minute) these are rough indicators that you are highly stressed. Feeling cold is another symptom, due to the suppressive effect of stress on the thyroid gland.

Supported by knowledge of how you feel and any stress-related symptoms, you can find out just where you stand in relation to stress which is one of the most common reasons for chronic fatigue. The chart below shows typical symptoms and test results for each stage of stress.

	Stage 0	Stage 1	Stage 2	Stage 3
	No stress	Normal stress	Prolonged stress	Chronic stress
		Normal response	Poor adaptation	Can't adapt
DHEA	Normal	High	Low	Low
CORTISOL	Normal	High	High	Low
	No stress	Stressed	Stressed out	Can't cope
	Even energy	Energy OK	Always tired	Chronic fatigue
	Concentration good	Concentration OK	Poor concentration	Unclear thinking
	Mood good	Irritable	Anxiety and depression	Depression
	Sleep good	Sleep OK	Disturbed sleep	Always tired

REBALANCING YOUR STRESS

All the measures advised in earlier chapters will help restabilise your stress response: avoiding stimulants, avoiding sugar and refined foods, increasing your intake of low GI foods and eating them with protein, and supplementing key energy nutrients. Getting the right kind of exercise and sufficient sleep will also help (see Chapters 13 and 14).

However, there is more that you can do to speed your recovery, especially if you know where you are in the stress cycle. Go into any healthfood store or pharmacy and you'll see a wide variety of so-called natural remedies designed to boost energy and combat stress. There are herbs such as ginseng, guarana, ephedra and licorice. You may also come across adrenal glandular extracts. Many pharmacies sell sugar pills containing measured amounts of caffeine. This, of course, is what most fizzy drinks contain, as well as tea and coffee.

All of these raise cortisol levels and should be avoided (with the exception of ginseng) if you're in Stage 2, with already high cortisol levels. If you further raise your cortisol levels you will speed up your progression to Stage 3 – exhaustion. If, however, you are already exhausted, licorice may help, unless your cortisol levels are shown to be extremely high. Choose licorice powder in capsules, rather than eating a highly sugared licorice sweet. Licorice slows the break-down of cortisol, thus making it last longer.[7] Siberian ginseng is OK under any circumstances. While it can raise cortisol it seems to work as an 'adaptogen', helping you to adapt by stabilising the stress response.[8] If your DHEA level has been shown to be low in an ASI test, you should supplement DHEA to correct this imbalance, then retest to find out whether your normal levels have been restored. DHEA supplements are available over the counter in the US, but not in the UK. DHEA is best taken only under the guidance of a practitioner, backed up with actual measures of your DHEA status from ASI tests.

In summary, the fastest way to rebalance your stress hormones is to:

■ Have your stress hormone levels checked

- Under the guidance of a qualified medical practitioner, supplement licorice and Siberian ginseng.

- If your DHEA level is low consider supplementing DHEA to correct the imbalance, under the guidance of a qualified practitioner.

- Whatever stage of the stress cycle you are in, avoid adrenal stimulants, change your diet, take nutritional supplements, do the right kind of exercise, get enough sleep and change your lifestyle to reduce your stress level.

PART 2

TUNING UP YOUR SYSTEM

CHAPTER 8

DIGESTION – THE KEY TO VITALITY

There are many reasons for chronic fatigue and most of them involve digestion. While an insufficient intake of the right nutrients can cause fatigue, so can poor digestion and absorption. Some people eat healthy food but, for one reason or another, don't digest it properly and therefore don't get the nutrients they need for energy.

There's also plenty that can go wrong in the digestive tract which, if laid out flat, would cover a small football field. This surface area is what comes between the 100 tons of food we consume in a lifetime and our inner selves. Only certain chemicals are allowed through, a selection process policed by the bouncers of the immune system.

Prolonged stress (marked by high levels of cortisol and low levels of DHEA) shuts down this immune function. It's as if the bouncers go on strike. The bouncers are called IgA (secretory Immunoglobulin A); they line the digestive tract and their job is to protect us by keeping undesirable molecules out. As our IgA levels fall when we're under stress, we lose this protection, which results in large numbers of undesirable molecules entering our bodies. These stimulate an immune response, which is what allergies are all about and why people under chronic stress are more likely to develop food sensitivities.

Too much stress suppresses the immune system and encourages inflammation, setting the scene for gastrointestinal infections and inflammation. Our bodies always react to stress by diverting our resources towards producing energy for fight or flight, and away from things like digestion and immunity. This is why it is harder to digest food when you're under stress and why you are more at risk of getting a cold or flu.

Another reason why uninvited guests get through into the body is our inner skin, the wall of the digestive tract, becomes too permeable, a condition known as gastrointestinal permeability or 'leaky gut syndrome'. This can be aggravated by an infection, inflammation, bloating, or too much alcohol or use of non-steroidal anti-inflammatory drugs such as aspirin and antibiotics.

Once too many toxins and large molecules start 'gatecrashing' through the digestive tract, the body has to work overtime to detoxify and deal with them. Before long the body's ability to detoxify all the uninvited guests starts to weaken, resulting in compromised liver function. By this stage even the slightest increase in toxins results in a whole host of symptoms such as fatigue, drowsiness, headaches, body aches and inflammation.

For example, when we exercise, our muscles tend to produce a toxin called lactic acid which can make them a bit stiff the next day. This is no problem normally, but if a person's detox potential is poor, even a brisk walk can trigger symptoms. So too could a slightly larger meal than normal, or certain foods, especially those that are hard to digest. This whole chain of events is the most common cause of 'chronic fatigue syndrome', proving that digestion is more often than not the key to vitality. As a Harvard Medical School Professor once said, 'Having a strong stomach and a good set of bowels is more important to human happiness than a large amount of brains.'

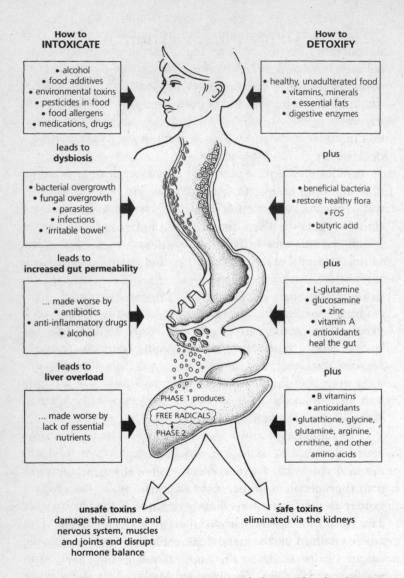

How to INTOXICATE

- alcohol
- food additives
- environmental toxins
- pesticides in food
- food allergens
- medications, drugs

leads to **dysbiosis**

- bacterial overgrowth
- fungal overgrowth
- parasites
- infections
- 'irritable bowel'

leads to **increased gut permeability**

... made worse by
- antibiotics
- anti-inflammatory drugs
- alcohol

leads to **liver overload**

... made worse by lack of essential nutrients

How to DETOXIFY

- healthy, unadulterated food
- vitamins, minerals
- essential fats
- digestive enzymes

plus

- beneficial bacteria
- restore healthy flora
- FOS
- butyric acid

plus

- L-glutamine
- glucosamine
- zinc
- vitamin A
- antioxidants heal the gut

plus

- B vitamins
- antioxidants
- glutathione, glycine, glutamine, arginine, ornithine, and other amino acids

PHASE 1 produces
FREE RADICALS
PHASE 2

unsafe toxins damage the immune and nervous system, muscles and joints and disrupt hormone balance

safe toxins eliminated via the kidneys

Figure 9 – How to intoxicate and detoxify the body

DIGESTING YOUR FOOD

You are not what you eat. You are what you can digest and absorb. The large food particles which we eat are broken down into tiny food particles that can enter the body (put on the guest list, so to speak). Carbohydrates are broken down into simple sugars such as glucose or fructose; proteins are broken down into amino acids; and fats are broken down into fatty acids and glycerol. At least that's what *should* happen.

The digesting is done by hydrochloric acid in the stomach and digestive enzymes. Each day the body produces around 10 litres of digestive juices and if you do not produce enough you will get indigestion. This can manifest as abdominal discomfort, bloating, excessive flatulence and fatigue. Instead of being energised by a meal you feel tired. Eating more than your body can digest can also bring on these symptoms.

If you suspect you might not be digesting your food very well the simplest way to check is to go to a healthfood shop and buy a digestive enzyme supplement (see Useful Addresses). Pick one that contains some amylase (the enzyme for digesting carbohydrate), some protease (the enzyme that digests protein) and some lipase (the enzyme that digests fat). Take one of these with each meal for a week. If you find your indigestion disappears and your vitality returns then you've hit the nail on the head. You can keep taking these digestive enzymes if you wish. However, more often than not, after a month they become unnecessary, especially if you've made the other dietary changes recommended in this book.

The reason for this is that enzymes are themselves dependent on vitamins and minerals. Stomach acid, for example, needs zinc to be made by the body. If you're not digesting properly you don't get the nutrients you need to make the enzymes to digest your food – it's a vicious circle. On the other hand, once you're digesting, you can take in more of the nutrients that help your body make more enzymes. That's why you can often stop taking the enzymes after a month and maintain the improvement. There is, however, no harm whatsoever in taking them on an ongoing basis.

BACTERIA IN THE BALANCE

Inside your digestive tract are no less than 3lb (1.3kg) of 300 different strains of bacteria which are essential for your health and vitality. If you take a course of antibiotics it more or less wipes them out, which is why you feel tired. These bacteria make all sorts of nutrients for the body and protect the digestive tract from infection.

Of course, there are harmful bacteria too, which you may have encountered on holiday or when you have had food poisoning. Having the right balance of bacteria is the key to digestive health and overall well-being. The symptoms of an imbalance are much the same as those discussed above for indigestion. If the digestive enzymes don't help, you may wish to consider increasing your intake of these beneficial bacteria. This is especially important if you've been doing anything that would tend to destroy them, such as drinking too much alcohol or taking antibiotics.

There are two ways to give your beneficial bacteria a boost. One is to eat fermented foods that contain the right strains of live bacteria. The two most prominent strains in the digestive tract are called Lactobacillus acidophilus and Bifido bacteria. Some 'live' yoghurts are cultured with these strains, so you could eat these. Most supermarkets sell 'live' yoghurts – check the sides of pots for which strains have been used.

An alternative is to take a 'probiotic' supplement. This is the name given to concentrated supplements containing beneficial bacteria. Again, look for those containing both Lactobacillus acidophilus and Bifido bacteria. The process of making such probiotic supplements is complex and needs careful control. The bacteria don't last forever. It is therefore best to choose a product from a reliable supplement company, keep them in the fridge and use them within six months of purchase (see Useful Addresses).

UFOs OF THE INTESTINES

More insidious than bacterial imbalances is UFO infestation. Unidentified faecal organisms (or UFOs) are the various harmful organisms that can take up residence in the digestive tract, including harmful bacteria, fungi, protozoa and worms. These parasites are far more common than is generally realised.

Symptoms of infection can include:

- abdominal pain and cramps
- diarrhoea and constipation
- bloating
- flatulence
- foul-smelling stools
- inflammatory gut problems
- fatigue
- headaches
- food sensitivity
- weight loss
- aches and pains
- fever

This list is by no means comprehensive and illustrates how UFO infestation could underlie many health problems. If you have developed symptoms after being on holiday in a 'high risk' area or perhaps after a course of antibiotics (which wipe out your natural defences against other parasites), then UFO infestation is a possibility.

The best course of action is to check by having a comprehensive stool test. There are many different kinds of parasites and the best laboratories test for a wide variety, the presence of beneficial and harmful bacteria, and the common fungal infection, Candida albicans. If you do have an infection then there are usually specific remedies to deal with particular parasites. This is a complex field and it is definitely best to go to a clinical nutritionist or medical specialist, who can get the appropriate test done for you (see Useful Addresses).

LEAKY GUT SYNDROME

We are designed to digest our food into simple molecules that can readily pass through the digestive tract and into the bloodstream. However, if a person doesn't digest their food properly, or if the gut wall becomes leaky, incompletely digested foods can enter the blood unheeded. There they are likely to alert immune 'scout' cells which treat them as invaders, triggering an allergic reaction. The ensuing battle results in a complex of chemicals that themselves are toxins and need to be cleaned up to be safe.

The gut wall can become leaky for a number of reasons, in addition to a suppressed immune system and low IgA. For example, alcohol irritates the gut lining, as does a protein in wheat, called gluten; a deficiency of cell-building nutrients, like vitamin A, zinc, protein and essential fats, can result in a poor gut wall structure; an overgrowth of the wrong bacteria or fungi, such as Candida albicans, or any other parasite, can burrow into the intestinal wall, irritating it and causing increased permeability; even abdominal distention, either as a result of bloating or over-eating, can overstress the gut wall. Certain drugs are also particularly damaging to the digestive tract. These include antibiotics, aspirin and other anti-inflammatory drugs.

Once the gut wall is permeable, perfectly normal foods can become toxic to the body because they gain access before being completely digested. Instead of increasing your energy level, these foods add to the toxic burden of the body and, once this is too great, the body can no longer satisfactorily detoxify itself. The resulting toxins can generate all sorts of symptoms, discussed in detail in the next chapter.

There are simple, non-invasive tests to find out if you have leaky gut syndrome (see Useful Addresses). These involve drinking certain substances and later collecting a urine sample. Depending on what appears in the urine, it is possible to define precisely what size molecules are passing through the digestive tract. These tests are best done under the guidance of a clinical nutritionist who can then devise a specific diet and supplement programme to heal the digestive tract. These often include specific supplements of butyric acid, I-glutamine and glucosamine which help to heal the digestive tract, as well as the vitamins and minerals listed below.

Whether or not you have leaky gut syndrome, in order to keep your digestive tract in good health, you need to:

- Avoid alcohol or have it infrequently and in moderation.

- Avoid taking aspirin or other non-steroid anti-inflammatory drugs on a regular basis.

- Cut down your intake of wheat, especially yeasted breads, and switch to oatcakes, wholegrain rye bread, and buckwheat pasta instead.

- Eat fermented foods such as live yoghurt, or take a probiotic supplement.

- Eat seeds and fish. The essential fats they contain are used structurally in the digestive tract, and act as natural anti-inflammatory agents.

- If you are suffering from indigestion try taking a digestive enzyme supplement with each main meal.

- Make sure your supplement programme includes 15mg zinc and 10,000iu (3300mcg) vitamin A, plus a high strength multivitamin including vitamin E (400mg) and vitamin C (1000mg).

CHAPTER 9

TESTING YOUR DETOXIFICATION POTENTIAL

Eating the right food is one side of the coin, detoxification is the other. It's all too easy to think that food is good for you. Of course it is, but the truth is that almost all food contains toxins as well as nutrients. So, too, do air and water.

THE CRUCIAL ROLE OF THE LIVER

From a chemical perspective, much of what goes on in the body is reasonably simple – substances are broken down, built up and turned from one thing into another. A good 80 per cent of this involves detoxifying potentially harmful substances. And much of this work is done by the liver which represents a clearing house, able to recognise millions of potentially harmful chemicals and transform them into something harmless or prepare them for elimination. It is the chemical brain of the body – recycling, regenerating and detoxifying in order to maintain our health.

These external or exo-toxins represent just a small part of what the liver has to deal with. Many toxins are also made within the body from otherwise harmless molecules. Every thought, every breath and every action can generate toxins. These internally created or endo-toxins have to be disarmed in just the same way as exo-toxins do. Whether a substance is bad for you depends as much on your ability to detoxify it as on its inherent toxic properties. Those with multiple food sensitivities are eating the same food as healthy people – they just have less detoxification potential.

Instead of thinking of certain substances as being 'bad' for you, or provoking allergies, think of them as exceeding your capacity to detoxify them. It's as if the body's metabolism represents a fire. The fire generates smoke that needs to be got rid of. Our metabolic fire (the consequence of using energy from the sun stored in plants) burns slowly and generates plenty of smoke. That's what the liver has to deal with – it's the smoke, not the substances themselves, that often causes problems.

RECOGNISING LOW DETOX POTENTIAL

Chronic fatigue syndrome (formerly known as ME, Epstein Barr and yuppie flu, among numerous other spurious titles) is a classic case of symptoms that don't fit into any conventional medical model. With no real method of diagnosis or treatment, many sufferers have been told it's all in the mind and have just been prescribed anti-depressants.

Yet chronic fatigue, multiple allergies, frequent headaches, sensitivity to chemicals and environmental pollutants, chronic digestive problems, muscle aches, autism, schizophrenia, drug reactions and Gulf War syndrome are just some of the conditions that may be caused by a breakdown in the body's ability to detoxify.

After spending years studying the symptoms associated with impaired detoxification potential, Dr Jeffrey Bland from the Functional Medicine Research Center in Gig Harbor, Washington, USA, developed the Metabolic Screening Questionnaire with common symptoms that indicate a low detox potential. Below is an abbreviated list of these common symptoms. If you have many of these symptoms the chances are that your ability to detoxify is impaired.

Do You have Low Detox Potential?

Score one point for every symptom you occasionally have, and two for those you have frequently.

Head	headaches; faintness; dizziness; insomnia
Eyes	watery or itchy eyes; swollen, red or sticky eyelids; bags or dark circles under the eyes; blurred vision
Ears	itchy ears; ear ache; ear infection; drainage from ear; ringing in ears; hearing loss
Nose	stuffy nose; sinus problems; hay fever; sneezing attacks; excessive mucus formation
Mouth	chronic coughing; gagging; frequent need to clear throat; hoarseness; loss of voice; swollen or discoloured tongue, gums or lips; ulcers
Skin	acne; hives; rashes; dry skin; hair loss; flushing or hot flashes; excessive sweating
Heart	irregular or skipped heartbeat; rapid or pounding heartbeat; chest pain
Lungs	chest congestion; asthma; bronchitis; shortness of breath; difficulty breathing
Digestion	nausea or vomiting; diarrhoea; constipation; bloated feeling; belching; passing gas; heartburn; intestinal/stomach pain
Joints/Muscles	joint/muscle aches or pain; arthritis; stiffness or limitation of movement; feeling of weakness or tiredness
Weight	binge eating/drinking; craving certain foods; excessive weight; compulsive eating; water retention; underweight
Energy	fatigue; sluggishness; apathy; lethargy; hyperactivity, restlessness
Mind	poor memory; confusion; poor comprehension; poor concentration; poor physical coordination; difficulty in making decisions; stuttering or stammering; slurred speech; learning disabilities
Emotions	mood swings; anxiety; fear; nervousness; anger; irritability; aggressiveness; depression

If your total score is above 25, you could have a detox problem and you should clean up your diet.

If your total score is above 50 your detox potential is definitely under par.

If your total score is above 75 you should seek the help of a nutritionist or medical practitioner.

If you have a significant score it's well worth going one step further and having your liver's detoxification potential tested. Fortunately, modern science has developed a non-invasive test that involves ingesting a measured amount of caffeine, aspirin and paracetamol and then analysing certain chemicals that appear in the urine. How these substances are dealt with, and what they turn into, shows how well each aspect of liver detoxification is working.

These comprehensive detoxification tests are available through doctors and clinical nutritionists (see Useful Addresses). They are, however, quite different from standard tests for liver function which involve measuring levels of key enzymes GPT and GOT. If these are raised, it means your liver is really struggling. This indicates a chronic problem and, while it is useful in pinpointing that a problem exists, it doesn't really identify the best way to help recovery.

DETOXIFICATION – A TWO-STAGE PROCESS

Our detoxifying mechanisms, mainly situated in the liver, are a complex set of chemical processes that can recycle toxic chemicals and turn them into harmless ones, in a process known as 'biotransformation'. Each detoxifying process (or pathway) consists of a series of enzyme reactions, and each enzyme is dependent on a number of nutrients that, step by step, make our internal world safe to live in.

Detoxification can be split into two stages. The first, known as Phase 1, is akin to putting your rubbish in bags, ready for collection. It doesn't actually eliminate anything, just prepares it for elimination, making it easier to pick up. Fat-soluble toxins, for example, become more soluble. Phase 1 is carried out by a series of enzymes called P-450 enzymes. The more toxins you're exposed to, the faster these enzymes must work to pile up rubbish ready for collection. Often, the substances created by the P-450 enzyme reactions are more toxic than before.

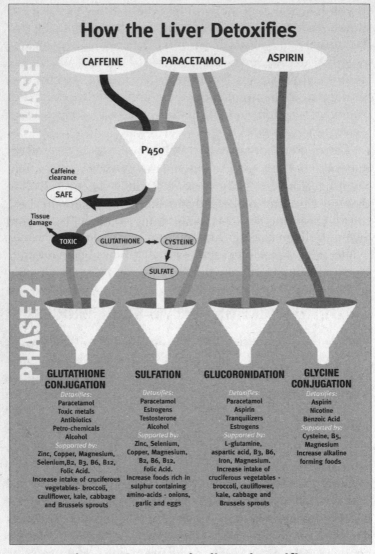

Figure 10 – How the liver detoxifies

The function of P-450 enzymes depends on a long list of nutrients, including vitamins B2, B3, B6, B12, folic acid, glutathione, branched chain amino acids (leucine, isoleucine, valine), flavonoids and phospholipids, plus a generous supply of antioxidant nutrients (vitamins A, C and E etc.) to deal with the oxidants.

Often a person who has a high exposure to toxins (perhaps due to diet and lifestyle factors or digestive problems) has a revved-up Phase 1 – their P-450 enzymes are used to working hard and fast to get these toxins ready for collection. Substances that get Phase 1 going include caffeine, alcohol, dioxins, cigarette smoke, exhaust fumes, high-protein diets, organophosphate fertilisers, paint fumes, saturated fat, steroid hormones and charcoal barbecued meat.

The second phase, known as Phase 2, is more about building up than breaking down. According to Dr Sidney Baker, an expert in the chemistry of detoxification, around 80 per cent of all the building the body does is for the purpose of detoxification.

The end-products of Phase 1, for example, are transformed by 'sticking' things on to them in a process called conjugation. Some toxins have glutathione stuck to them (this is called glutathione conjugation). This is how we detoxify paracetamol (acetaminophen), for example. In cases of overdose, a person is given glutathione to mop up the highly destructive toxins generated by Phase 1 detoxification of this drug.

Other toxins have sulphur stuck to them in a process called sulphation. This is the fate of many steroid hormones, neurotransmitters and, once again, paracetamol. The sulphur comes directly from food. Garlic, onions and eggs, for example, are good sources of sulphur-containing amino acids such as methionine and cysteine so if you lack these you've got a problem. Others have carbon compounds, called methyl groups, stuck to them (this is called methylation). Lead and arsenic are detoxified in this way. Aspirin has the amino acid glycine stuck to it (called glycine conjugation). When these pathways are overloaded the body can use another, known as glucuronidation, which is the primary route for breaking down many tranquillising drugs.

TOO MANY TOXINS OR NOT ENOUGH NUTRIENTS?

When these biochemical pathways don't work properly, due to overload or a lack of nutrients, the body generates harmful toxins. One example is homocysteine, a toxic by-product of breaking down the amino acid methionine. This can be a result of problems with sulphation (usually due to a lack of vitamin B6), or methylation (which needs folic acid). Sulphur dioxide, a component of exhaust fumes, is detoxified via the sulphation pathway whose enzymes depend on the mineral molybdenum, which is particularly high in beans. Over-exposure, coupled with a molybdenum-deficient diet, can lead to intolerance of exhaust fumes.

These detoxifying pathways work together. If one is over-loaded a toxin may be processed by another. But, once the back-up systems are overloaded, the body is unable to clear toxins which can then damage and disrupt just about every system in the body, including the nervous system, hormone balance, muscles and joints, digestion and immunity. The collection of symptoms that develops goes under many names, but the most common is chronic fatigue syndrome.

In summary, lack of energy and decreased ability to cope with stressors (physical, psychological and chemical) can result from an impaired ability to rid the body of harmful toxins – both those taken in from the outside and those generated from normal body processes. To find out if this is a factor for you:

- Test your detox potential using the questionnaire on p. 72.

- If your score is significant consider seeing a clinical nutritionist and having a comprehensive detoxification test.

The next chapter explains how to detoxify your body and give your energy levels a boost.

CHAPTER 10

DETOX NOW AND BOOST YOUR METABOLISM

For centuries, health experts have extolled the virtues of spring-cleaning the body. In much the same way as you need a holiday from work, your body needs a break from detoxifying. One of the traditional methods of purifying the body is fasting. The fact that many people report feeling so much more vital after fasting is testimony to the fact that making energy is as much about improving the body's ability to detoxify as it is about eating the right foods.

However, not everybody immediately feels better as a result of fasting. It is quite common for people to experience a so-called 'healing crisis' when they feel worse for a few days and then feel better. What we are learning about detoxification suggests that some of these people may be experiencing a real crisis, rather than a healing crisis. Once the body starts to liberate and eliminate toxic material, if the liver isn't up to the job symptoms of intoxication can result. Modern detox regimes therefore tend to use modified fasts, in which the person is given a low-toxin diet, plus plenty of the key nutrients needed to speed up the body's ability to detoxify. Doing this once a year, for a couple of weeks, can make a major difference to your energy levels.

Alternatively, a more focused approach would involve consulting a clinical nutritionist and having a comprehensive detoxification profile test. On the basis of your results they will devise a specific diet and supplement programme designed to restore optimal detoxification potential. I have seen many long-term sufferers of chronic fatigue syndrome completely recover within weeks of implementing such a nutritional programme. And I am convinced that the vast majority of people with chronic fatigue syndrome can be helped in this way.

THE TWO-WEEK DETOX DIET

Obviously, the first step towards detoxifying the body is to remove or lessen the toxic load. Some foods are nearly all toxin-generating, while others are nearly all detoxifying. Most, however, have good factors and bad factors.

Good Detox Foods

All fruits and vegetables are definitely good for detoxification. They should make up the bulk of your two-week detox diet. Needless to say, you should choose organic wherever possible so your body doesn't have to detoxify the pesticides.

Fruit

The most beneficial fruits with the highest detox potential include: fresh apricots, all types of berries, cantaloupe, citrus fruits, kiwi, papaya, peaches, mango, melons and red grapes; go easy on bananas (one a day only); dried fruit is best avoided during these two weeks.

Vegetables

All vegetables are great but these are especially good: artichokes, peppers, beetroot, Brussels sprouts, broccoli, red cabbage, carrots, cauliflower, cucumber, kale, pumpkin, spinach, sweet potato, tomato, watercress; white potatoes and avocado should be eaten in moderation; also excellent are sprouted beans and seeds (try alfalfa, sprouted mung beans, chick peas, lentils, aduki beans and sprouted sunflower seeds – available ready-sprouted in most healthfood shops and some supermarkets and green grocers).

Low-Toxin Foods

The following foods are generally good for you, but may contain low levels of toxins. These should make up no more than a third of your two-week diet.

Grains   Brown rice, corn, millet, quinoa.

Fish   Salmon, mackerel, sardines, tuna.

Meat   Organic skinless chicken, turkey and wild game.

Oils   Use extra-virgin olive oil for cooking and in place of butter, and cold-pressed seed oils for dressing (organic, cold-pressed flax oil is best for this).

Nuts and seeds   Have a large handful of raw, unsalted nuts and seeds each day (try grinding them up and sprinkling them over a fruit salad; include almonds, brazils, hazelnuts, pecans, pumpkin seeds, sunflower seeds, sesame seeds and flax seeds).

Foods to Avoid on Your Detox Diet

The following foods, while normally OK in moderation, are best avoided during your two-week detox diet because they are either hard to digest, mildly irritate the gut or are hard to detoxify.

Gluten grains   Barley, oats, rye and wheat (including spelt and kamut).

Meat and dairy produce   Milk and all dairy products, eggs and organic red meat.

Harmful Foods and Pollutants

The following foods and pollutants should be avoided at all times:

Red meat, refined foods (e.g. white bread/pasta/rice, sugar and any foods containing it), salt and any foods containing it, hydrogenated or partially hydrogenated fat, artificial sweeteners, food additives and preservatives (a good general rule – if you can't pronounce it, avoid it!).

Alcohol, tea, coffee and all fizzy drinks including cola drinks and squash.

Also avoid as far as possible fried foods, pesticides, exhaust fumes and medications – most contain harmful substances that require detoxification.

Detox Drinks

During these two weeks alcohol is obviously out. It is a major toxin for the body. So too are any sources of methylxanthines, a family of chemicals that includes caffeine, tannin, theobromine and theophylline. This means no chocolate, coffee or tea, and no peppermint tea either.

Alternatives include:

- Fruit juice – Always dilute with an equal quantity of water.
- Aqua Libra, Ame and Elderflower Champagne for special occasions!
- Herbal teas – There is now a huge variety to choose from. Sample a few until you find the one you like best.
- Rooibos tea – caffeine-free and tastes very similar to 'normal' tea.
- Dandelion coffee – Can be drunk as a coffee replacement while you are on your two-week detox diet. Once it is complete, try Caro, Barleycup or Teecino.

The best drink of all is pure water and lots of it. Drink 2 litres of purified, distilled, filtered or bottled water a day. This may seem an awful lot, but water puts no burden on the body and helps to dilute toxins as they are eliminated.

Detox Supplements

Supplementing the nutrients that help the body to detoxify is a great way to speed up the benefits of this rejuvenating diet. The nutrients needed to support the first stage (Phase 1) of detoxification are vitamins B2, B3, B6, B12, folic acid, glutathione, branched chain amino acids, flavonoids and phospholipids, plus a good supply of antioxidant nutrients to disarm dangerous intermediary oxidants created during this phase. For guidance on nutrient amounts refer to the levels given for individual nutrients in Chapter 19.

Phase 2 of detoxification can be stimulated by a specific list of nutrients including the amino acids glycine, taurine, glutamine and arginine. Cysteine, N-acetyl cysteine and methionine are also precursors for these nutrients (i.e. the body can convert these into the others).

You can help support the detoxification process by supplementing the following, as well as by sticking to the two-week detox diet recommendations.

All twice a day
Multivitamin and multimineral
Antioxidant
Vitamin C 1000mg
Rejuvan (glutathione and anthocyanidins) 1 (not with food)
l-glutamine 2000mg (not with food)
Milk thistle 100mg

See Useful Addresses for suppliers.

If you suspect that your energy problem may be connected with detoxification follow this regime for two weeks and see how you feel. Alternatively, consult a clinical nutritionist, have a comprehensive detoxification profile test, and follow the specific diet and supplement programme your nutritionist designs on the basis of your test results.

CHAPTER 11

....

SOLVING CHRONIC
FATIGUE SYNDROME

While fatigue is an incredibly common symptom (reported by 15 to 30 per cent of patients consulting their doctors), severe chronic fatigue syndrome, formerly known as ME, is much rarer, probably affecting less than 1 per cent of patients. It is, however, very much on the increase. Chronic fatigue syndrome didn't officially exist until 1997 when a joint report published by the Royal Colleges of Physicians, Psychiatrists and General Practitioners abandoned the term 'myalgic encephalomyelitis', meaning inflammation of the sheath of nerve cells in the brain, and agreed to call the condition chronic fatigue syndrome (CFS); they did admit, though, that they were still baffled as to its cause and the best form of treatment.

CFS may not be a new condition – it bears many similarities to vaguely defined syndromes, both epidemic and sporadic, described in the medical literature since the late eighteenth century. It also has much in common with a Victorian condition known as neurasthenia, a syndrome in the US called Chronic Epstein–Barr virus (the agent that causes glandular fever), ME, depression, fibromyalgia, allergies, multiple sclerosis, auto-immune disorders and pesticide exposure. Victims of Gulf War syndrome – now thought to be the result of massive exposure to organophosphate pesticides, coupled with the effects of nerve gas protection tablets – also show the same pattern of health problems.

In the US the condition is diagnosed in cases where severe fatigue halves activity for at least six months and is not caused by any other recognisable illness. Sufferers would also need to exhibit eight out of eleven of the following symptoms: mild fever, recurrent sore throat, painful lymph nodes, muscle weakness, muscle pain, prolonged fatigue after exercise, recurrent headache, joint pain, psychological complaints, sleep disturbance and sudden onset of symptoms.

WHAT CAUSES CFS?

Exactly what's behind the apparent increase in CFS cases remains a bit of a mystery.

While there appears to be no single underlying cause, it is common for CFS sufferers to have disturbed immune system function and the presence of an infectious agent and/or Candida albicans, a type of fungus that can inhabit the digestive tract. If Candida is present, it can be treated using an aggressive nutrition-based strategy based on starving the organism of sugar, while building up the healthy gut bacteria, boosting the immune system and taking antifungal agents.

Another candidate for the infection theory is the Epstein-Barr virus. However, too many cases of CFS test negative for this virus for it to be a likely cause; it may instead be an opportunist, taking advantage of CFS sufferers whose immune systems have been weakened.

NUTRITIONAL DEFICIENCY

One of the greatly overlooked factors in CFS is nutritional deficiency. The usual assumption is that if you eat a well-balanced diet you get all the nutrients you need, yet scientific studies have shown significant improvement by giving CFS patients magnesium, vitamin B12 or essential fats (both evening primrose oil and fish oil combinations). Deficiency of many nutrients, including B vitamins and vitamin C, results in fatigue and one very real possibility is that those with CFS have especially high requirements for certain nutrients. Of all the nutrients so far tested, the most consistently beneficial is the mineral magnesium.[1]

The most likely possibility is that CFS is a product of 21st-century living – with its combination of poor diet, 'anti-nutrient' exposure and overuse of drugs. Anti-nutrients encompass a range of substances that deplete nutrients from the body, or heighten the body's need for them: from lead exposure and chemicals in detergents to alcohol and pesticides. All these factors, plus infections, may be enough to overload the body's defences, resulting in CFS.

While conventional medics may be at a loss to explain this condition, nutritionists have pioneered a highly effective treatment using a combination of diet and supplements, designed to improve gut and liver function and boost immunity. This approach is based on a new understanding of the sequence of events that leads to CFS. Imbalances in digestion and absorption are usually involved, resulting in gut dysbiosis and infection with unfriendly bacteria, fungi or other pathogens. This can be followed by increased gut permeability, leading to allergies and immune reactions, which cause the liver's detoxification systems to become overloaded. An infection may often trigger CFS, or it can be the result of a gradual weakening of the gut, liver and immune systems.

EVIDENCE OF DETOXIFICATION PROBLEMS

Dr Jeffrey Bland and his colleagues at the US Institute of Functional Medicine tested 30 CFS patients for liver detoxification abnormalities (as described in Chapter 9), and then devised a nutritional strategy to correct these. Using the Metabolic Screening Questionnaire (an abbreviated form of which appears on p. 72), the initial symptom score over the

21 days of the study dropped by more than half, from 173 to 77 points;[2] this was consistent with improvements shown by further liver function tests. In later research they found that a significant proportion of CFS patients had a particular type of imbalance in liver detoxification in which the first phase was very speedy, generating toxins, while the second phase was sluggish, resulting in an inability to clear toxins.[3] This indicates the great importance of people with CFS having their liver function assessed and treated using specifically designed nutritional support.

Other factors that may be involved are food allergies (often caused by leaky gut syndrome), adrenal exhaustion, thyroid problems and blood sugar problems, which have been discussed in earlier chapters.

In conclusion, CFS is a very real condition that may represent an advanced state of imbalances that, in more minor forms, account for the widespread incidence of less severe fatigue. The best explanation of the symptoms to date is that the body fails to adapt to a set of circumstances that may include sub-optimum nutrition, chronic stress and exposure to toxins, as well as poor digestion, poor detoxification, hormonal imbalances and immune dysfunction. The most effective treatment involves a tailor-made diet, backed up by specific supplemental nutrients, based on proper evaluation of these factors by a clinical nutritionist.

PART 3

ENERGY SAVERS

CHAPTER 12

ELIMINATING THE ENERGY EXPENDERS

There are two sides to the energy equation: one is generating energy; the other is conserving it. We consume the energy available to us in many ways and often get 'burnt out'. All stressors and stimulants can be thought of as energy consumers. The 'high' is literally energy leaving the system, like a wave that breaks and seems, for a few seconds, to be full of energy. A few seconds later there is no wave at all – the energy is gone.

One of the models I have found most useful for understanding how and why we do things that deplete our energy is described by the psychologist and philosopher Oscar Ichazo, founder of the Arica Institute and originator of the Protoanalytical theory. In an article on drug abuse he says:

> Drugs (all of them) can be characterised as 'energy consumers', consuming energy at a rate much greater than our natural ability to replace it. As drugs burn all our accumulated vitality in short periods of time, the brief exaltation is inevitably followed by depletion of vital energy, felt as the 'down', the depressant effect of drugs. Nothing can replace a natural, clean body capable of producing natural and clean vital energy.

He rates the drugs most damaging to our vital energy in this order: alcohol, heroin and opiates, tobacco, cocaine, barbiturates, anti-depressants, amphetamines, marijuana and caffeine.

His model, called the Doors of Compensation®, describes the nine different ways we dissipate energy – stimulants and drugs are just one of these. Compensating in one way or another is completely natural and can be seen as the means by which we keep ourselves psychologically in balance. Think of our consciousness – the psyche – as a container. When we react emotionally to situations, when things don't go the way we expected, when we experience stress in one form or another, the pressure in our psyche increases. To release the pressure we use one or more of the Doors of Compensation. That's why, for example, people go boozing on Friday night, or take it out on the family by being bad-tempered, or stuff themselves full of food. These are all ways of dissipating energy and reducing the psyche's tension.

THE DOORS OF COMPENSATION®

Understanding how we use these Doors of Compensation® helps us to identify sources of stress and enables us to develop healthier ways of staying in balance. This process is the purpose of a one-day training course presented by sponsors of the Arica Institute (see Useful Addresses) which is a tremendous tool for dealing with stress.

The Doors of Compensation® include:

1. toximania   the use of toxic substances including cigarettes, alcohol and cannabis

2. psychosomatic illness – being over-preoccupied with one's mental and physical health and illness

3. over-exertion – which might manifest as workaholism or excessive exercise

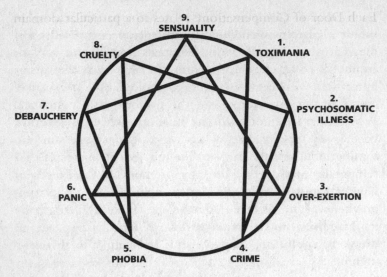

The Doors of Compensation®

4. crime – ways of getting even because you don't feel you got a fair deal

5. phobia – from dislikes to aversions

6. panic – always being in a panic and then spreading it to others

7. debauchery (excess) – which could manifest as excessive intake, for example of food

8. cruelty – which includes being mean, and using abusive language and behaviour

9. sensuality – which includes excessive sex and over-preoccupation with the pleasures of the senses.

Each Door of Compensation® relates to a particular domain where a specific psychological imbalance occurs. For example, when we have stress in the work domain we go into panic. So, having the objectivity to notice which 'doors' are attractive to you also shows the aspects of your life where you are generating internal pressure.

While we all use these ways of compensating at different times every day, the degree to which we use them is also significant. The first degree of use is just occasionally, for temporary satisfaction. For example, the odd occasion you have a couple of drinks after a stressful week. The next degree is when you drink every day and you are anaesthetised by it. The third degree is when you habitually drink, with drunkeness as the outcome, which is debilitating. By this stage such behaviour amounts to a level of addiction and represents a continual dissipation of energy.

FOODS AND DRINKS TO AVOID

From the point of view of nutrition, the foods and drinks that are associated with dissipating energy, if used regularly or habitually, are sugar, alcohol, coffee, tea and chocolate. To generate and maintain a good level of energy it is best either to avoid these completely, or at least to get to the point where they are an occasional treat and not a daily prop.

Another way of dissipating energy is to eat too much. Indian lore says we should fill our stomachs with one half food, one quarter water and leave one quarter for the 'prana' or vital energy. This means, eat to the point where you are satisfied, but not full. This has the effect of energising you, while overeating has the opposite effect.

So, nutritionally, it is best to avoid all the energy consumers and not overeat. This will certainly give you more energy to deal with stress in your life. However, from the psychological point of view, these 'doors' are used for a purpose – to relieve internal pressure. So, if you deal with the issues that generate the psychological pressure, your need to use energy-depleting third degree Doors of Compensation® will be reduced. In other words, you need to change the way you react as well as changing what you eat and drink – the two go hand in hand.

CHAPTER 13

OXYGEN, BREATHING AND EXERCISE

From a chemical point of view there are two things you need to produce energy – glucose and oxygen. Oxygen is really the most important nutrient of all. About 80 per cent of the human body is made from it and it is part of water, fat and protein. Oxygen deficiency causes death in minutes. The assumption is that we all get enough from breathing, yet there is a big difference between 'enough' and 'optimal levels'. It is also important to remember that there are many factors in air apart from oxygen. A few hours spent breathing city air, compared to mountain air, will provide a vivid example of how air quality can affect your vitality.

ARE YOU GETTING ENOUGH OXYGEN?

New Zealand scientist Dr Les Simpson believes that chronic fatigue syndrome and muscle pain can often be the result of a lack of oxygen. Oxygen is required by all cells for metabolism. It is carried around the body in the arteries by the red blood cells. As the arteries become narrower and narrower, turning into tiny blood capillaries, the red blood cells release the oxygen so that it can pass through the capillary wall into the surrounding cells. At the capillary–cell interface, the cell receives oxygen and nutrients from the blood, and gives off carbon dioxide and other unwanted by-products of metabolism.

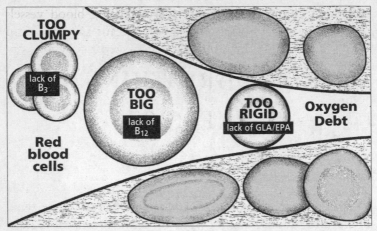

Figure 12 – Nutrients that help deliver oxygen

These capillaries are only 4 microns wide, yet red blood cells are typically 8 microns in diameter. How, wondered Simpson, do they pass along such a narrow space? The answer is, they squeeze through. Yet some red blood cells are too large, others are too inflexible and some clump together. These can create a 'log-jam' which results in a poor oxygen supply to cells, resulting in a build-up of lactic acid and poor cell function. One tell-tale sign of chronic fatigue is muscle pain after exertion. The symptoms of muscle pain also occur in polymyalgia, an increasingly common diagnosis, particularly among older women. A number of researchers have also observed a lack of oxygen in the frontal lobes of the brain, in people diagnosed with schizophrenia.

So, what's the answer? A lack of B12 is the most common cause of over-sized red blood cells, while a lack of essential fatty acids makes them too rigid and unable to squeeze through. Niacin (vitamin B3) can also help by increasing the electrochemical charge on cells so that they repel each other and don't clump together, as well as dilating blood vessels through the release of histamine (which causes a short-term blushing effect). If this problem is suspected, it can be corrected by supplementing 100mg or more of niacin twice a day, essential fats GLA 150mg (Omega 6) and EPA 500mg (Omega 3), and vitamin B12 10mcg. Vitamin B12 is usually included at this level in a multivitamin.

ENERGY OUT OF THE BLUE

Assuming you've got all the nutrients you need to deliver oxygen efficiently, is there any point in taking in even more? The answer is 'yes', although too much oxygen is also dangerous. Critically ill people are sometimes put in oxygen tents. Within complementary medicine there is a whole speciality, known as oxygen therapy, devoted to ways of enhancing oxygen balance in the body. However, there are things you can do right now to increase your ability to use oxygen.

Most people use less than one-third of their lung capacity. Physical and breathing exercises all increase use of lung capacity, thereby helping to oxygenate the tissues and improve energy levels. The best forms of exercise in this respect are aerobic, stamina-building activities like swimming, jogging, exercise classes, cycling and brisk walking, which all require you to breathe deeper and harder. Deep breathing is beneficial in all forms of exercise. Time the movements with the breath, pay attention to it and breathe from your stomach, as this helps to open up the rib cage, allowing more air in.

THE BREATH OF LIFE

Breathing is something we take for granted and yet, for thousands of years, ancient traditions have used breathing exercises to promote conscious, healthful changes in the body. Our breathing is a reflection of our emotions. Each emotional state has its own distinct breathing pattern. For example, when we are anxious or afraid, our breathing becomes rapid and shallow. Conversely, when we are happy and at ease our breathing is naturally slow and deep. Working with the breath is a fundamental part of meditation and yoga. The breath is said to link the mental and physical – it is the key to calming the mind and relaxing the body.

What's more, by slowing and deepening your breathing, you may actually live longer. Man's quest for longevity has thrown up numerous theories as to the secret of slowing the ageing process. Yet only one statistic remains consistent. All animal species have, on average, 2.5 to 3.5 billion heartbeats in a life. For man, with an average heart rate of 72, the average lifespan is 70 to 80 years. By this equation, slowing your heart rate to 60 beats per minute would add seven years to your lifespan. Deeper breathing and a slow pulse are recognised signs of health. The stronger your heart, the less often it needs to beat; and the deeper the breath, the more tissues can be oxygenated. But there may be more to breathing than that. As well as containing oxygen, according to yoga philosophy the air we breathe also contains 'prana', or vital energy. By doing conscious breathing exercises we can accumulate this energy and revitalise the body and mind.

THERE'S MORE TO AIR THAN OXYGEN

Science is moving ever closer to measuring this invisible energy. Some scientists think it's connected with charged particles in the air, called ions. When these particles are negatively charged they have positive effects on us – and vice versa. This is what ionisers are all about. They generate negative ions.

High levels of positive ions, the bad guys, are found during strong winds, such as the Mistral that blows along the Rhone valley in France. With it comes the equivalent of PMT (Pre-Mistral Tension), as the wind is rumoured to make you grumpy and irritable. After a thunderstorm, or close to a waterfall, the air is charged with negative ions, the good guys. These may literally help you accumulate vital energy.

If you don't happen to have a waterfall close by, doing specific breathing exercises will have a similar effect. Most yoga and meditation techniques (see below and Chapter 15) teach specific ways to deepen your breathing. This is not only good for oxygen delivery, but also a great way to calm your emotions, and clear your mind. Tension makes the breath shallow, while deepening the breath reduces tension.

ENERGY EXERCISE

Energy isn't just about the food you eat and the air you breathe. It also depends on the state of your body. Without exercise your body loses muscle tone, it accumulates tension and you feel tired. Exercise improves your circulation and oxygenates your blood, which increases your energy level. But there's more to exercise than simple physical training.

Scientific research into yoga and T'ai Chi has identified a positive health effect that can't be gained from aerobics classes or running around the park. While excessive aerobic exercise can actually depress the immune system and overstress the body (though for most of us over-exercise is not the issue!), T'ai Chi can boost well-being and immunity. Yoga has been shown to have positive effects on pulse, blood pressure,[1] and mental and physical performance, beyond those expected from physical exercise alone.

These ancient systems of exercise were never designed simply to make us fit. They were designed to generate vitality by removing the blockages caused by accumulated tension. Such blockages prevent vital energy (an invisible ingredient, known in China as 'chi') from restoring our vitality.

Every day we accumulate stress. This is stored in our minds as anxiety and in our bodies as tension. The underlying philosophies of the Eastern martial arts and the ancient Indian traditions all teach that tension blocks the flow of vital energy, and stops us being rejuvenated. Therefore the purpose of doing yoga or T'ai Chi is to release the blocks, unlock the tension and allow us to return to a state of equilibrium. Of course, while they may help you maintain a level of fitness, develop some strength and stay supple, yoga and T'ai Chi can hardly be described as 'aerobic'. Nor are you likely to end up looking like Demi Moore or Bruce Willis.

PSYCHOCALISTHENICS

Enter Psychocalisthenics, developed by Oscar Ichazo, founder of the Arica Institute in New York, an organisation dedicated to helping people achieve their full potential. He based his exercise system on the premise: if you're going to spend 20 minutes a day getting fit, you might as well generate vital energy at the same time. Psychocalisthenics, a routine of 23 exercises that can be done in less than 20 minutes, is a complete contemporary exercise system which, at first glance, looks like a powerful combination of yoga, dance, T'ai Chi and martial arts. 'In the same way that we have an everyday need for food and nourishment we have to promote the circulation of our vital energy as an everyday business,' says Ichazo, a master of martial arts and yoga. He first developed Psychocalisthenics in 1958 and it has since been tried and tested by thousands of people.

Psychocalisthenics means strength (*sthenia*) and beauty (*cali*) through the breath (*psyche*). The breath is the driving force in this routine, as each of the 23 exercises is guided by a precise deep breathing pattern. This combination of movement, breath and exercises, designed to generate vital energy, is what makes Psychocalisthenics unique – a perfect combination of

East and West. When I first did the routine, (which takes a day to learn) I was amazed at how light and re-energised my body felt afterwards. My muscles felt tuned and my joints more flexible, but the major benefit was the feeling of clear-headedness.

Other advocates of Psychocalisthenics (shortened to Psychocals) give the same glowing reports. 'This is exercise pared to perfection. I wasn't sweating buckets as I would after an aerobics class but I could feel I had exercised far more muscles. I was feeling clear-headed and bright rather than wiped out,' said Jane Alexander, when she reviewed the routine for the *Daily Mail*. In the US, Psychocals is now promoted by the 'Bionic Woman', actress Lindsay Wagner.

One of the things I like most about Psychocals is that you don't have to go anywhere, or wear special clothes, or buy any equipment. Once you've learnt the routine you can do it in 16 minutes in your own home, accompanied either by the video, or with a 'talk through' music tape.

The best way to learn it is to do the one-day training, held frequently in different locations throughout Britain (see Useful Addresses). You can learn it from the video, but there's nothing like having someone there to tell you what you're doing wrong and how to do it right. There's also a fascinating book called *Master Level Exercise*, which explains the theory behind Psychocals and how each exercise revitalises different parts of the body and mind.

REDEFINING VITALITY

Vitality, the very real experience of feeling full of energy, is more than just a consequence of your diet and physical fitness. The extra factor is the one that's harder to measure, but no less tangible. Vital energy (called 'chi' or 'ki' in the East) is described as the energy we draw in from the universe and, depending on how receptive we are, it has the power to nourish us at a fundamental level.

As mentioned above, yoga, T'ai Chi and other martial arts are all designed to make us more receptive; so too is acupuncture, which works by unblocking channels of energy (called 'meridians') through which this vital energy is said to flow. When you walk by the ocean, lie on a beach, or stroll through a forest you feel more 'connected', more 'in touch'; and this gives you renewed vitality and a different perspective on life. Vital energy is that hidden ingredient that connects us with each other and with the world around us.

According to traditional Chinese medicine, vital energy comes to us from the food we eat and the air we breathe. I am convinced that this is more than just the sum of the nutrients in our food and the effects of oxygen or negative ions alone. Eating organic, fresh foods, prepared consciously, has, I am sure, a profoundly different effect to eating fast food, such as a hamburger, made from grossly mistreated animals, and reconstituted fries, made from pesticide-laden potatoes: this cannot be explained by their nutrient content alone. Similarly, I believe that it isn't just *what* we breathe, but *how* we breathe it, that nourishes us.

In summary, to maximise your overall energy and resistance to stress, you need to:

- Include some form of de-stressing exercise, such as Psychocals, yoga or T'ai Chi, in your weekly routine.

- Be conscious of your breathing and learn how to breathe deeply as a means of reducing tension and as a centring technique. Each of the above exercise systems teach breathing exercises.

- Spend as much time as you can in clean air. If you are a city-dweller, choose holidays in the mountains or by the ocean and go for walks in the country.

CHAPTER 14

THE POWER OF SLEEP

Sleep provides essential nourishment for both the body and the mind. People who are stressed often have sleep-related problems, while a lack of sleep is itself a stress factor. When we first go to sleep the brain waves goes through various stages, effectively slowing down. The most regenerative stage for the body is when the brain's signals are in slow wave formation. This usually occurs during the first 90 minutes of sleep and then at intervals during the night. After about 90 minutes the brain goes into another phase, known as Rapid Eye Movement (REM) sleep. It is thought that this phase is associated with dreaming and is particularly important for psychological health and well-being. It goes without saying that if you don't get enough sleep, REM or not, the consequence is fatigue.

The effects of sleep are far-reaching on your health. Both too little and too much are associated with an earlier death. Statistically the amount of sleep that correlates with the longest lifespan is between five and nine hours a night. Particularly as we age, there is a higher correlation between few (less than five) and great (more than nine) hours of sleep and increased mortality. Seven hours sleep is linked to the lowest death rate.[2] Just as important is the quality of sleep – many people, as they age, have more fragmented and light sleep and don't get enough time in slow wave or REM sleep.

SLEEP AND THE BODY

During the night, and especially during these slow wave and REM phases, the brain produces higher levels of growth hormone, also known as somatotrophin. This hormone helps with the repair and replacement of tissue and bone. During the daytime growth hormone levels are lower. When you're stressed, the subsequently high levels of the stress hormone cortisol further suppress growth hormone, diverting energy away from repair into coping with the energy demands of a stressful situation.

Normally, when you are asleep cortisol levels are low. But at times of chronic stress cortisol levels may not drop sufficiently while you sleep. This further suppresses tissue repair, effectively speeding up the ageing process. Although not yet proven in research, the dynamics of sleep and stress suggest that it's best to go to sleep unstressed. If this is so, late-night horror movies are out. Instead do something relaxing to help you get a good night's sleep.

How you wake up is important too. Normally, cortisol and adrenalin levels are lower during the night. Consequently, your pulse rate and blood pressure should be lower when you wake up and increase when you get up. If you wake with a fast pulse rate or high blood pressure, and then, when you stand up, there is no further increase, this is indicative of high cortisol levels during the night. This kind of 'desynchronisation' does occur in some people and is thought to be part of the dynamics of seasonal affective disorder and other forms of depression. Under these circumstances it is best to see a clinical nutritionist who can run a 24-hour salivary hormone test to find out what's out of sync and make recommendations to bring everything back into balance.

Another cause of high blood pressure and increased pulse rate on rising is a condition called apnoea, which is thought to affect between 3 and 8 per cent of men. This is when a person's breathing is somewhat abnormal during the night, resulting in the improper exhalation of carbon dioxide, and thus insufficient oxygen. Apnoea is more common in people who snore and can be brought on by going to sleep after drinking alcohol. Stress may also contribute to this condition which, in turn, is associated with fewer REM phases and therefore less restorative sleep.

SLEEP AND THE MIND

As far as the mind is concerned, the most critical phases of sleep are the bursts of REM sleep. These tend to last for about 30 minutes, occurring, on average, five to seven times a night. If a person is deprived of REM sleep they don't feel fully rested on waking and are more likely to get depressed. When they do get a chance to sleep they have longer periods of REM sleep. All this suggests that our minds need to have this time while we're asleep to process what's been happening in our lives. It is generally thought that we dream during these phases and that dreams are important for mental and emotional health. Once again, high levels of the adrenal hormone cortisol mean less REM sleep. Some anti-depressants have the effect of suppressing REM sleep – one wonders what effect that has on a person's psychological state.

TREATING SLEEP PROBLEMS

Often stress is accompanied by difficulty getting to sleep or staying asleep. Both can be the result of poor nutrition or the effect of too much stress and anxiety on the nervous system. Calcium and magnesium have a tranquillising effect, as does vitamin B6. Tryptophan, a constituent of protein, has the strongest tranquillising effect and, if taken in doses of 1000mg to 3000mg, is highly effective in treating insomnia. It takes about an hour to work and remains effective for up to four hours.

In the same 'family' as tryptophan is 5-hydroxytryptophan which is available in healthfood stores; it is approximately ten times more potent so a dose of 100 to 300mg is recommended. While tryptophan is non-addictive and has no known side-effects, its regular use is not recommended – it is better to adjust your lifestyle so that no tranquillising agents are needed. Tryptophan turns into the important brain chemical serotonin, sufficient amounts of which are important for proper sleep and normal brain function.

Another common stress-related sleep problem is 'restless legs', a condition where a person can't settle down and keeps wanting to move their legs. This is known to be linked either to drinking coffee at night or deficiency in zinc and iron. Once again, optimum nutrition and following all the advice in this book about cutting back on stimulants and alcohol will help promote a good night's sleep.

In summary, to get maximum benefit from sleep, you need to:

- Make sure you get between six and eight hours of uninterrupted sleep a night.

- Avoid stimulants and alcohol, especially after 6 pm.

- Go to bed in a relaxed frame of mind.

CHAPTER 15

MEDITATION AND THE MIND

As good food is to the body, meditation is to the mind. Studies on meditation have shown that the positive effects are greater than those gained simply from sleep.[3] These include increased peace and contentment, better responsiveness to stressful events and quicker recovery from them, reduced heart rate and blood pressure, slower rate of breathing and more stable brain wave patterns. Meditation has also been shown to prevent the depression of the body's immune responses that usually occurs with stress.[4] People who practise meditation on a regular basis have been found to be less anxious and there is little doubt that meditation and relaxation techniques are effective in dealing with anxiety, stress and insomnia.[5]

However, the true power of meditation in generating energy, clarity and peace goes beyond the beneficial effects that have been measured in clinical studies. No one would doubt that stress is a mental, as well as a physical phenomenon. The true power of meditation is the way it helps us gain control over the mind. According to the fourth-century psychologist, Patanjali, through meditation, 'The mind can be used to undo the mind.'

This has tremendous significance for those so habitually stressed that even the mildest conflicts generate an exaggerated stress reaction more appropriate for dealing with a life-threatening situation. For such people meditation can be the way to 'unlearn' this conditioned stress response and become less reactive to the normal conflicts that life presents.

FOCUSING THE MIND

The starting point for meditation is focusing your thoughts on one object, be it a sound, a candle flame or your own breath. By concentrating on a single point, the power of the mind seems to grow and, with that, your mental energy intensifies. This is the opposite of what happens when you are stressed and exhausted, when your mind tends to flit from one thing to another, leaving a trail of panic and confusion.

I became interested in meditation when, as a psychologist, I was researching the effects of nutrition on mental performance. We had shown that the non-verbal IQ scores of children could be raised simply by giving them a multivitamin and multimineral supplement. But what exactly was the reason for this? Later studies showed that the children who were taking vitamins weren't cleverer as such than those who weren't taking them. It was just that they were more focused and consequently could answer more questions in the allotted time. It is this focusing ability that is crucial.

As I started to meditate on a regular basis I found that my mind became quieter and I was able to focus on the task at hand, instead of dissipating my energy by trying to do many things at the same time and not really doing any of them properly. However, even this benefit is superficial compared with what happens at deeper levels of meditation.

THE TRUE GOAL OF MEDITATION

With time and good instruction, those who meditate find they slip into an elevated state of awareness, a kind of pure 'being' in which the mind is naturally still, the body relaxed and the emotions settled. This state is real, not imagined, and correlates to a distinctive change in brain wave patterns. After such a meditation, your energy, mental clarity and ability to stay unaffected by the turbulence of daily life, are significantly greater.

There is, however, still more. Even these stages of deep meditation are merely preparation for the ultimate goal of meditation in which the full power of the mind and true vitality available to each one of us become apparent. This highest state of awareness is described by Patanjali, a fourth-century Indian sage, as 'Diminishment of mental fluctuations, like a precious or clear jewel assuming the colour of any object.' The fruit of meditation is a state in which the difference between subject and object melts away. Often described as a sense of unity or connectedness, it marks the end of life as a struggle or 'fight'. While the 'fight–flight stress response' may help us survive in a hostile world, I believe there comes a time in life when it is possible to live without conflict and to draw on the full power of the vital energy that is available to each and every one of us.

While many have tasted these states of mind, few live in them permanently. For this reason, as part of your action plan for dealing with stress and maintaining a high energy level, you should set aside time for meditation each day in whatever form that takes for you. For some this means walking the dog; for others listening to music or having a bath with aromatherapy oils; or perhaps taking some time for contemplation, prayer or meditation. If you would like to learn how to meditate, there are courses available – see Useful Addresses.

CHAPTER 16

MANAGING YOUR TIME

Time is precious. Poor use of it is a major source of stress and waste of energy, yet time management is a vital skill not taught in schools. I have been particularly, impressed with the work of Michael Walleczek in this area. (An ontologist with a primary interest in organisational transformation, he acts as a consultant, has advised many leading organisations (from BMW to Nike). Walleczek's work fits in well with what is known about mental performance and nutrition. Once again, the underlying theme is focus and attention. Nutritional intervention studies have proved that optimum nutrition improves mental performance by increasing concentration and attention span.

'The sense of being overwhelmed is a consequence of having unfinished business,' says Walleczek. This certainly struck a chord with me, as I was always armed with endless 'to do' lists that would run through my mind like a frantic record. I would often end up spending my day doing things other than the things I was supposed to be doing. Isn't that crazy – to be worrying about the things you're not doing, while doing something else!

In fact, the only time that actually exists is now – the present. As one saying I like goes, 'The past is history, the future a mystery. Now is the only time there is. It's a gift. That's why we call it "the present".' Being able to stay focused in the present is the hallmark of truly efficient and effective people. What is the difference between these two qualities – efficiency and effectiveness? 'Efficiency is doing the thing right, while effectiveness is doing the right thing,' says Walleczek.

To do the thing right is to do it completely. To have it done and dusted. Isn't it having a whole lot of things going on, each at an incomplete stage, that generates stress? Isn't it part of human nature to want to solve problems, resolve conflicts and complete tasks?

Yet, how often do we start something else before finishing the thing we were doing? The nature of the human mind is such that it is only able to focus on one thing at a time. Our attention can flit rapidly from one thing to another. However, in every moment, the mind can only have one point of focus, in the same way that we can only have one field of vision.

Fully realising the truth of this is the beginning of developing effective time management. The first step for me was to gather together all my piles of papers, bills to pay, things to read, projects to look at, things to do, and to decide, one by one, am I really going to do this? And, if so, when?

I went to the stationer's and bought a 'time management system' – a concertina file, with compartments labelled 1 to 31 for the days of the month, and some clear plastic folders. As I picked up each pile of papers I would decide if and when I was going to deal with it. Much got thrown away, and the papers that were left were each put in a plastic folder, allocated to a space in time. Now, as I start each day, I know what I am doing and I have all the paperwork I need for the task at hand. I have days when I pay my bills, days when I catch up on reading or do my correspondence, and 'catch up' days, when I file all those little things that are not urgent.

Instead of being surrounded by piles of paper and endless

'to do' lists, I now have everything filed according to the time I've allocated to deal with it. If that time is not today then I don't think about it. As a result of working in this way I get more done in less time, with a substantial reduction in stress.

Many people feel increasingly overwhelmed by the apparent demands of modern living. Our world is changing rapidly. Advances in technology are making the world smaller and the speed of change faster. There is a continual explosion in information on every subject. Our choices as to how to live, what to eat, where to go, what to buy are multiplying equally rapidly. It's a new world and we need new tools to help us adapt to the fast pace of modern life. Parts 1 and 2 of this book aim to give you nutritional tools to help your body adapt to a chemical environment that includes your food, water and air. They also enhance your adaptive potential so that you can respond to inevitable stress in a way that allows you to stay in equilibrium.

The psychological and organisational tools that help you to adapt to today's world are equally important. While these are not specifically the subject of this book, you may want to consider developing these skills – by attending courses, reading books and seeking advice – as part of your action plan for high-energy living.

PART 4

THE ENERGY EQUATION

CHAPTER 17

ACTION PLAN FOR HIGH-ENERGY LIVING

If you not only want to survive but to thrive in the twenty-first century you need to make an investment in you. Nothing has a more significant effect on your life than your energy. With a good energy level you can respond to new opportunities, deal skillfully with stressful situations, enjoy life and take advantage of the many joys of this world. Your state of energy is not fixed at birth. It isn't genetic. It depends on how you live and what you eat and drink. The energy equation is a combination of changes in your lifestyle and your diet, plus supplements.

This book contains more than enough information to make a big difference, whatever your particular circumstances may be. What follows is a finely tuned daily routine, designed to get the best out of you. You may not feel you can apply it all in one go, nor that you can fulfil all the requirements every day. However, it will give you a clear idea of what to aim for and how to adjust your current diet and lifestyle.

'Man is a knackered ape', a schoolchild once said in an exam howler. Our fellow men and women are no exception; most have learned to prop themselves up with sugar and stimulants and live in a permanent state of stress. Now, however, is your chance to 'unlearn' these habits. This means breaking with tradition, be it coffee and croissants on Saturday morning or boozing on Friday night. Instead, you have the opportunity to become part of a new culture of people fully equipped to face the future with energy and enthusiasm. Few people turn back, once they have tasted the difference between feeling 'just alright' and feeling positively vital.

In 1977 I undertook an experiment similar to the one I'm suggesting for you. Out went the stimulants, sugar and alcohol (or, at least, most of it), and in came masses of fruit, vegetables, wholefoods and supplements. Within a fortnight I was experiencing a level of energy and mental clarity that I had never known before.

I used to wake under a cloud and head, on remote control, for the kettle to make a strong cup of coffee. Instead, a few days after starting my new routine I was waking as if under a clear, blue sky, fully alert and ready to start a new day. My mind seemed sharper and my concentration improved dramatically. By the end of the first month I knew I never wanted to feel like I used to. Although it took me years to incorporate everything into my daily life, now what I want to eat is what's good for me. I still enjoy delicious food and drinks and, for the most part, choose those that will enhance my health.

THE 12 GOLDEN RULES

These golden rules will help you increase your resistance to stress and enable you to maintain a high energy level:

- Avoid sugar and high-Gl foods, instead eating low-Gl foods. Generally, combine carbohydrate-rich foods with protein-rich foods to lower the Gl effect of the meal (see Chapter 3).

- Eat foods rich in the 'energy nutrients' – vitamins B, C and Co-Q, magnesium, calcium, zinc and iron (see Chapter 4).

- Take a high-strength multivitamin and multimineral, providing significant amounts of B vitamins, plus extra vitamin C and chromium (see Chapter 4).

- Stop using stimulants on a regular basis – tea, coffee, ciga-rettes, chocolate and caffeinated drinks (see Chapter 5). If you smoke, quit, following the guidelines in Chapter 6.

- Follow the 20-day detox diet twice a year to improve your detoxification potential, and generally follow a low-toxin diet (see Chapter 10).

- Identify how you expend energy, not just with alcohol or coffee, but with other Doors of Compensation®, such as over-exertion, gluttony or cruelty. Consider what it is you are compensating for and develop better ways to respond and deal with stressful situations (see Chapter 12).

- Include some form of de-stressing exercise in your weekly routine, such as Psychocals, yoga or T'ai Chi (see Chapter 13).

- Be conscious of your breath and learn how to breathe deeply as a means of reducing tension and as a centring technique.

- Spend as much time as you can in clean air. If you are a city-dweller choose holidays in the mountains or by the ocean and go for walks in the country (see Chapter 13).

- Get enough sleep, ideally seven hours a night, undisturbed (see Chapter 14).

- Put aside some time for meditation, contemplation or get-ting away from it all (see Chapter 15).

- Learn how to manage your time effectively (see Chapter 16).

If you are very stressed or exhausted, have your stress hor-mone levels checked and, on professional recommendation, supplement adaptogens such as ginseng or licorice to restore normal stress response (see Chapter 7). If you suspect you have digestive or detoxification problems see a clinical nutritionist and consider having a comprehensive detoxification test (see Chapters 8 and 9).

What all this means, in terms of what you eat and what you supplement, is explained in the next two chapters.

ESTABLISHING A DAILY ROUTINE

The key to putting all this into practice is to establish a daily routine. Of course, the exact prescription is different from one person to another, so you need to identify what it is that makes the biggest difference for you and what works in terms of your daily timetable and other commitments. The key is your morning routine. What you do in the first hour of every day often sets the tone for the whole day. Here's my ideal morning routine.

Morning

Psychocalisthenics or run in the park	15 minutes
Shower	10 minutes
Meditation	15 minutes
Breakfast	15 minutes

When I'm writing I get up earlier and snack on a piece of fruit before starting this amazingly energising one-hour morning routine.

Midday

During a working day it's important to have a break at lunchtime, even if it's just for half an hour. You will digest your food much better if you don't eat in a state of stress, with adrenal hormones pumping. It also gives you a chance to appreciate what you are eating and to chew it properly, rather than gulping it all down in seconds.

Afternoon

After work it's a good idea to do something that changes the energy from work to relaxation. This is a great time, for example, to go for a walk or a jog, or do yoga or T'ai Chi, meditate, listen to music or read a good book.

Evening

Eat dinner early so there's at least two hours between finishing the meal and going to sleep. Make sure the last thing you do before going to sleep is to relax. Maybe watch something light on TV (not the news), or read and listen to music. The important thing is not to go to sleep in a state of stress.

CHAPTER 18

High-Energy Food

The foods to eat for high energy are the foods that can be most efficiently turned into energy in the body. In the early days of nutritional science it was thought that sugar – effectively pure body fuel – would be the best energy food. However, we now know that a high-sugar diet lacks the micronutrients needed to turn it efficiently into energy and, because it is so 'high-octane', it disrupts blood sugar levels.

Today the search is for 'miles per gallon' – discovering which foods allow the human body to function efficiently, with stable blood sugar control, and an ideal all-round supply of the many nutrients involved in maintaining consistent energy. Not surprisingly, this line of enquiry has led us right back to the very foods we evolved to eat – unrefined, organic, nutrient-rich wholefoods, with an emphasis on lots of vegetables and fruit.

THE HIGH-VITALITY DIET

Eating for vitality means:

• Avoiding refined sugars, including honey.

• Avoiding refined carbohydrates, including white bread, biscuits, cakes, white rice and other processed foods.

- Avoiding coffee, tea and cigarettes.

- Limiting alcohol.

- Eating more vegetables, raw or lightly cooked. Aim for four servings a day.

- Having three pieces of fresh fruit a day.

- Eating more beans, lentils, nuts, seeds and wholegrains.

- Unless you're vegetarian, eating fish and free-range chicken instead of meat.

- Drinking plenty of water, herb teas or diluted, unsweetened fruit juices.

These foods help you maintain sufficient blood sugar levels for consistent energy and avoid peaks and troughs in blood sugar levels which stimulate the release of stress-related hormones. It's best to eat high-GI carbohydrates (see Chapter 3) together with some protein; and to graze, not gorge. In other words, eat three meals a day with two snacks, rather than only having one or two large meals.

For vegetarians, and indeed anyone wanting to promote their health, it's best to balance your intake of carbohydrate from fruit and vegetables by eating plenty of 'seed' foods. For any seed to grow it must be rich in protein, plus a host of other key nutrients. Seed foods include: beans, soya produce, tofu, lentils; wholegrains such as oats, quinoa, wholewheat, rye, barley, brown rice, buckwheat; nuts and seeds such as almonds, sesame, sunflower, pumpkin and flax seeds.

Putting this into practice would mean, for example:

- **For breakfast,** having a wholegrain cereal containing its seed or germ, such as oat flakes with some ground seeds and fresh fruit with milk or soya milk. Such a breakfast provides plenty of low-GI carbohydrate, together with protein.

- **For lunch,** a wholegrain rye bread sandwich with tuna and loads of vegetables (watercress, lettuce, tomatoes, etc). Again, this would provide low-GI carbohydrates with protein.

- **For dinner,** a tofu and vegetable steam-fry, served with wholewheat or buckwheat pasta would again provide low-GI carbohydrates with plenty of protein from the tofu and a small amount from the wholegrain pasta.

- **For mid-morning snacks,** a couple of pieces of fruit, perhaps with a few almonds, or a couple of oatcakes or a carrot with some hummus.

Chapter 20 gives plenty of examples of how to put these principles into practice. And there are lots more recipes in my book, *The Low-GL Diet Bible*. These recipes and menus are all consistent with eating for energy, although the quantities are less important for those not wishing to lose weight.

THE 'WHEN' AND 'WHAT' OF EATING FOR ENERGY

When you eat is as important as what you eat. The most important meal of the day is breakfast. Many people skip breakfast or have a cup of coffee and a piece of toast.

Yet what you eat for breakfast determines how you feel for the rest of the morning. It is, however, also a mistake to eat so soon after surfacing that your digestive system is not yet fully functioning. If you start your day with 15 minutes of exercise your appetite will soon swing into action. Then it is time for a decent breakfast, as described above.

What you eat during the day depends on your lifestyle. A diet high in fruit and vegetables is simply not as filling as our traditional high-fat, high-protein diet. This means you may need to snack on fruit mid-morning and mid-afternoon.

Studies comparing the effects of eating little and often, compared to a couple of large meals a day, consistently show better health for those who 'graze' rather than gorge.[1]

If your day is stressful it is better to have a light lunch that requires little digestion, but, most importantly, to get out of the office, put your feet up and stop thinking about work even if it's only for 15 minutes.

You need at least two hours to complete the first stage of digesting a meal so dinner should never be later than two hours before the time you go to sleep. If you haven't given up all stimulants yet, do avoid tea and coffee after 6 pm.

CHAPTER 19

SUPPLEMENTS FOR SUPERCHARGE

Nutritional supplements, taken on a regular basis, make a big difference to your overall energy level. Even if your diet did provide all the RDAs of nutrients, these levels are way below those needed for maximum vitality. The better you feel, the more easily you can deal with stress. Also, the more stressful your life, the more nutrients you need. The advice in this book aims to maximise the amount of nutrients you can get from your diet and make up the shortfall through a sensible, balanced use of nutritional supplements.

If you are sceptical about nutritional supplements you have nothing to lose except your scepticism by trying this supplement programme for one to three months. Nutrients in supplement form are neither dangerous nor toxic, nor do they create 'dependencies'. They are simply concentrated food nutrients in pill form. Often the doses that produce results are many times higher than the levels found in food. Some people become unduly alarmed by this, although there is no need to. A tenfold increase in dietary intake of most nutrients leads to no more than a doubling of available nutrients to the cells. So relatively large amounts need to be taken to saturate cells with these vital energy catalysts, thereby maximising cell efficiency. What's more, the body knows how to deal with excesses, perhaps with the exception of fat-soluble vitamins A, D, E and K in very large quantities.

The chart below shows the ideal daily intake of each nutrient in supplement form, assuming a reasonable diet. The **basic** level is recommended for everybody to maintain a basic level of good health. The **high energy level** is for people wanting maximum energy or who are under a lot of stress. The **supercharge** level is the maximum one should take for up to one month to restore very low energy levels.

Supplements for Supercharge

Nutrient	Basic	High energy	Supercharge
B1	25mg	50mg	100mg
B2	25mg	50mg	100mg
B3	50mg	100mg	150mg
B5	50mg	100mg	200mg
B6	50mg	75mg	100mg
B12	10mcg	50mcg	100mcg
Folic Acid	100mcg	200mcg	400mcg
Biotin	50mcg	100mcg	150mcg
Co-Q10	10mg	30mg	90mg
Vitamin C	1000mg	2000mg	3000mg
Calcium	150mg	300mg	500mg
Magnesium	100mg	200mg	300mg
Iron	5mg	10mg	15mg
Zinc	10mg	15mg	20mg
Chromium	100mcg	200mcg	300mcg

This long list of nutrients is best obtained by supplementing your diet with the following:

Basic
2 to 3 × high-strength multivitamin and multimineral
1 × vitamin C 1000mg

High energy

2 to 3 × high-strength multivitamin and multimineral
2 × vitamin C 1000mg
1 × chromium 200mcg
1 × Co-Q 30mg

Supercharge

2 to 3 × high-strength multivitamin and multimineral
1 × high-strength B complex
3 × vitamin C 1000mg
1 × chromium 200mcg
1 × Co-Q 90mg

The foundation of any supplement programme is a good, high-strength multivitamin. Look for one that at least meets the basic needs for B vitamins and has 50–100mcg of chromium. The good ones say 'take two or three a day' because you simply can't get these amounts of nutrients into one tablet. One of my favourites is Solgar's VM 2000 (see Useful Addresses).

Co-Q is sometimes included in B complex formulas, usually at a level of 10–30mg. If you buy it separately, Co-Q supplements in an oil-soluble form are best absorbed. They usually come in 30 and 90mg strength.

The most common dosage of chromium is 200mcg. My preferred supplement form is chromium polynicotinate, which is chromium bound to vitamin B3.

There are optional extras, such as ginseng and licorice, but these depend on your stress hormone status. Also, for those with detoxification problems, there are many nutrients that help improve your detoxification potential. Guidance on these, however, is best given by a clinical nutritionist who can make a comprehensive, individual assessment of what you need.

Supplements, being food nutrients, are best taken with

food; preferably with breakfast or at lunchtime. The cost of such a programme is in the order of 40 to 50p a day – less than the price of a cup of coffee, a glass of wine, five cigarettes or a packet of crisps and a bar of chocolate. Most people start to experience the benefit of a supplement programme within 30 days, although the initial benefit is really best judged after three months. For optimal health and energy, supplements should be taken every day on an on-going basis.

CHAPTER 20

HIGH-ENERGY BREAKFASTS, LUNCHES AND DINNERS

To help you put all this into practice, here are seven daily menus designed to give you energy. By following these recipes for vitality and taking the supplements recommended in Chapter 19, you are likely to experience an improvement in your energy within a week. Sample daily menus are given first, followed by the recipes. You can make up your own menus by switching the individual breakfasts, lunches and dinners around, based on what you like the most; you could also devise your own meals based on the principles in Chapter 18.

HIGH-ENERGY MENUS

DAY 1
Breakfast: Fruit Muesli (p. 131) or Get Up & Go (p. 130)
Lunch: Cottage Corn Salad (p. 135)
Dinner: Fish Pie (p. 138) with Watercress Salad (p. 147)
Snacks: A piece of fruit with some almonds or a tablespoon of pumpkin seeds
Two oatcakes with hummus

DAY 2
Breakfast: Porridge (p. 131) or Get Up & Go (p. 130)
Lunch: Energy Sandwich (p. 133)

Dinner: Chilli (p. 139) with brown basmati rice and steamed
broccoli
Choice of dessert (pp. 149–152)
Snacks: A piece of fruit with nuts or seeds
Carrot and celery with hummus

DAY 3
Breakfast: Fruit Yoghurt (p. 132) or Get Up & Go (p. 130)
Lunch: Nutty Three-Bean Salad (p. 136) with Green Salad
(p. 146)
Dinner: Steam-fried vegetables (p. 140) with brown basmati rice
Snacks: A piece of fruit with nuts or seeds
Two oatcakes with hummus

DAY 4
Breakfast: Fruit Yoghurt (p. 132) or Get Up & Go (p. 130)
Lunch: Crunchy Tofu Salad (p. 136)
Dinner: Roast Vegetables with Quinoa (p. 141)
Choice of dessert (pp. 149–152)
Snacks: A piece of fruit with nuts or seeds
Carrot and raw broccoli with hummus

DAY 5
Breakfast: Fruit Muesli (p. 131) or Get Up & Go (p. 130)
Lunch: Energy Baked Potato (p. 134)
Dinner: Grilled Burger (p. 142) with rye bread and salad
Snacks: A piece of fruit with nuts or seeds
Two oatcakes with hummus

DAY 6
Breakfast: Scrambled Egg (p. 132) or Boiled Egg (p. 133)
with rye toast, or Get Up & Go (p. 130)
Lunch: Tofu and Avocado Dip with Crudités (p. 137) and
oatcakes

Dinner: Thai Baked Cod (p. 143) with brown basmati rice and Crunchy Thai Salad (p. 146)
Snacks: A piece of fruit with nuts or seeds
Carrot with hummus

DAY 7

Breakfast: Fruit Yoghurt (p. 132) or Get Up & Go (p. 130)
Lunch: Energy Soup (p. 137)
Dinner: Pesto Chicken (p. 143) with boiled new potatoes and steamed vegetables or Mediterranean Tomato and Broccoli Salad (p. 147)
Choice of dessert (pp. 149–152)
Snacks: A piece of fruit with nuts or seeds
Two oatcakes with hummus

RECIPES FOR VITALITY

If you equate healthy food with endless salads and boring bean dishes, these recipes will prove an extremely pleasant surprise. Each recipe is balanced to help keep your energy levels up.

Almost all the recipes are sugar-free, using the natural sweetness present in food. They are also high in fibre, so you don't need to add any extra. The foods used are naturally high in vital vitamins and minerals. And you should try to buy the freshest ingredients, organic if possible, since these tend to contain more nutrients, as well as being chemical-free.

As this diet is mainly based on fresh vegetables, fruits, beans, lentils and wholegrains, with some fish and chicken, you will find it very economical. You may, however, need to vary the fruits and vegetables, depending on what's in season.

All lunch and dinner recipes (except sandwiches and baked potatoes) are for two people unless otherwise stated.

Ingredients and Methods

Get Up & Go

Get Up & Go is a powdered breakfast drink made by blending skimmed milk or soya milk with a banana and a serving of Get Up & Go. Nutritionally speaking, it is the ultimate breakfast: each serving gives you more fibre than a bowl of porridge, more protein than an egg, more iron than a cooked breakfast, and more vitamins and minerals than a whole packet of cornflakes. In fact, every serving of Get Up & Go gives you at least 100 per cent of every vitamin and mineral and a lot more of some key nutrients. For example, you get 1000mg of vitamin C – the equivalent of more than 20 oranges.

Get Up & Go is made from the best-quality wholefoods, ground into a powder. The carbohydrate comes principally from apple powder; the protein comes from quinoa, soya and rice flour; the essential fats from ground sesame, sunflower and pumpkin seeds; the fibre from oat bran, rice bran and psyllium husks; and additional flavour from almond meal, cinnamon and natural vanilla.

It contains no sucrose, no additives, no animal products, no yeast, wheat or milk, and tastes delicious. Each serving, with ½ pint (300ml) skimmed milk or soya milk and a banana, provides less than 300 calories, making it ideal as part of any balanced diet. It is nutritionally superior to any other breakfast choice and is totally suitable for adults and children alike. It is fine to have this for breakfast every day, if you choose. It is my breakfast of choice – an excellent way to start the day if you lead a busy life. If you have a banana with it, choose a small one that is not too ripe. Low-GI alternatives are a soft pear or a heaped tablespoon of berries eg. raspberries, blackcurrants, strawberries (See Useful Addresses for stockists.)

Ground seeds

Some of the breakfast recipes include ground pumpkin and flax seeds. For this, you you should buy a packet of each at your healthfood store (flax seeds are linseeds). Mix them together in a glass jar and store them in the fridge. Each day, grind a spoonful in your now-redundant coffee grinder.

Quinoa

Quinoa is an excellent source of protein, as well as slow-releasing carbohydrate. It is said to have been the secret of the strength of the Aztecs who ate it as a staple food. It is a seed-like grain that you boil like rice, adding it to twice as much water so the grain can expand. It takes only 13 minutes to cook. The flavour is a bit like rice and it is best eaten as an accompaniment to, for example, a steam-fry or casserole. You could also add it to a soup to thicken it up, or eat it cold as part of a salad – much like couscous.

Tofu

In terms of protein quality, tofu is second only to quinoa – and is again an excellent source of protein and slow-releasing carbohydrate. Both tofu and quinoa, when eaten with carbo-hydrate-rich foods, slow down the release of their sugars. Tofu is the curd of the soya bean and is a bit like a bland cheese. It comes soft (good for desserts or making things 'creamy') or hard (better for steam-fries and main meals).

While its own flavour is quite bland, tofu can absorb the flavour of any sauce. So, for example, if you were cooking a Chinese steam-fry, flavoured with soy sauce, garlic and ginger, the tofu would take on this flavour and taste delicious. You can buy tofu already flavoured, such as smoked tofu, marinated tofu pieces and braised tofu, which make an excellent substitute for meat or chicken in steam-fries, stews and casseroles. These are firmer and more flavourful than plain tofu. You can also add flavour to tofu yourself by marinating it for 20 minutes. You can even include it in sandwiches. Always drain off the liquid in the packet first. Buy a brand which guarantees non-genetically modified soya, such as Cauldron Foods.

Steam-frying

One recipe refers to 'steam-frying'. This is quite different from frying or stir-frying, in that the ingredients are essentially steamed rather than fried. The lower temperature of steaming doesn't destroy nutrients to anything like the same extent as frying.

It is best to start with a shallow pan, or a deep frying pan, with a thick base and a lid that seals well. For a completely oil-free steam-fry, add 2 tablespoons liquid (either water or vegetable stock) or water down a fraction of the sauce you are going to cook with. Once this is almost boiling, add some vegetables, turn the heat up and put on the lid. The vegetables will sweat and start to cook. After a minute, add the rest of the ingredients. Turn the heat down after a couple of minutes and steam in this way until cooked.

Alternatively, start off by adding a fraction of olive oil, just to lightly coat the saucepan. Warm the oil and add the ingredients. As soon as they are sizzling, after a couple of minutes, add 2 tablespoons water or vegetable stock, or the sauce you are going to use, and cook with the lid on. In this way the vegetables can be 'steam-fried', using a fraction of the fat used in frying. The shorter the time you steam them for, the more taste the vegetables will have.

Breakfasts

GET UP & GO

½ pint (300ml) skimmed milk or low-fat soya milk
1 banana or pear or 1 heaped tablespoon berries
1 serving Get Up & Go (see Useful Addresses)

1. Blend milk, fruit and Get Up & Go powder until smooth, and serve.

FRUIT MUESLI

You can make this delicious muesli yourself. Experiment with different fruit combinations. It tastes best when the oats/rye are soaked overnight in enough water to cover them.

2 tablespoons oatflakes *or* 1 tablespoon oats and 1 tablespoon rye flakes
⅖ pint (220 ml) skimmed *or* soya milk
1 chopped apple, banana or pear *or* 1 heaped tablespoon berries
3 tablespoons natural yoghurt
1 dessertspoon ground flax and pumpkin seeds

1. Soak the oats/rye overnight.
2. Add the skimmed or soya milk.
3. Top with seasonal fruit, yoghurt and seeds.

PORRIDGE

On a cold winter's day nothing can be more warming than porridge. Oats are known to promote a healthy heart and arteries and they are full of fibre and complex carbohydrates.

½ pint (300ml) skimmed *or* soya milk
1oz (25g) porridge oats
1 teaspoon honey
1 dessertspoon ground flax and pumpkin seeds

1. Put ½ pint (300ml) water and half the milk in a saucepan and sprinkle in the oats.
2. Bring to the boil and boil for five minutes, stirring all the time.
3. Serve with the remaining milk, the honey and the ground seeds.

FRUIT YOGHURT OR YOGHURT SHAKE

Low-fat, live, natural yoghurt is a first-class food, unlike its commercial counterpart, in which most bacteria have been destroyed for a longer shelf life. Live yoghurt is packed with good bacteria that have a spring-cleaning effect on your digestive system, as well as being a fine source of protein.

5oz (125g) very low-fat, live yoghurt
1 teaspoon honey
1 chopped banana, apple, pear or kiwi *or* 1 heaped tablespoon berries
1 dessertspoon ground flax and pumpkin seeds

1. Combine all the ingredients, using any fruit that is in season, and serve.
2. If you prefer, make a shake by processing the mix in a blender.

SCRAMBLED EGG

While eggs are rather high in fat, as an occasional part of a balanced diet they are a good source of protein and add variety.

1–2 free-range eggs
dash of skimmed or soya milk
1 tablespoon chopped parsley
small knob of butter

1. Beat eggs with milk and parsley.
2. Melt butter in a small saucepan.
3. Pour in egg mixture. Cook slowly, stirring constantly.
4. Serve with wholegrain rye toast.

BOILED EGGS

This simple breakfast makes a wholesome start to the day.

1–2 free-range eggs

1. Boil the eggs to taste (3–4 minutes for soft-boiled).
2. Serve with wholegrain rye toast.

Lunches

ENERGY SANDWICHES

Fill two slices of rye bread or a wholemeal pitta pocket with any of the following combinations, and eat with a large portion of Coleslaw (p. 145) or Carrot Soup in the Raw (p. 145):

- cottage cheese and a large handful of alfalfa sprouts
- hummus, alfalfa and cucumber slices
- roasted chicken breast (skin removed) and sliced tomato
- smoked tofu, sliced tomato and watercress
- canned salmon *or* tuna in brine, cucumber and cress
- hard-boiled egg with cress, tomato and lettuce

ENERGY BAKED POTATO OR SWEET POTATO

Like a sandwich, a baked potato can be used as a great base for a satisfying lunch. A sweet potato makes a delicious change from the usual varieties. Remember to eat the skins, as they're full of fibre. When making your own, bake them for as short a time as possible, till they are cooked but firm on the inside. Have them with any of the fillings below and a large salad or Coleslaw (p. 145):

- canned salmon *or* tuna in brine, blended with 1 teaspoon cottage cheese
- low-fat cottage cheese with chives
- hummus with a handful of alfalfa sprouts
- baked beans
- Dahl (p. 144)
- roasted chicken breast (no skin) tossed in 1 tablespoon yoghurt dressing (blended with black pepper and fresh chives or mint)
- tofu tossed in 1 teaspoon tamari (a wheat-free type of soy sauce)

COTTAGE CORN SALAD WITH PUMPKIN SEED DRESSING

The combination of cottage cheese, corn and seeds increases protein quality as well as tasting delicious.

6oz (150g) low-fat cottage cheese
1 little gem lettuce, chopped
½ small green pepper, sliced
a handful of alfalfa sprouts
kernels cut from a raw corncob, *or* 4oz (100g) frozen corn, cooked very
   slightly
8 cherry tomato halves, to garnish

FOR THE DRESSING:
1 tablespoon ground pumpkin seeds
1 tablespoon low-fat natural yoghurt
1 teaspoon low-fat mayonnaise
1 teaspoon skimmed milk

1. Combine all the salad ingredients.
2. Mix together the dressing ingredients in a bowl.
3. Toss the salad in the dressing, and serve.

NUTTY THREE-BEAN SALAD

Beans are the best possible food for satisfying your appetite and giving you stamina.

12oz (300g) mixed beans (e.g. haricot, kidney and flageolet)
a handful of walnuts
chopped parsley to taste
2 tablespoons olive oil
2 teaspoons tamari *or* soy sauce
juice of 1 lemon
4oz (100g) fennel, chopped
4 spring onions, finely sliced
black pepper to taste

1. Combine all the ingredients and serve with a large, mixed salad.

CRUNCHY TOFU SALAD

This crunchy salad is one of my favourite lunches. It not only gives you a colourful variety of vegetables, but also a good helping of protein. Cauldron Foods' marinated tofu is available in most supermarkets.

12oz (300g) packet marinated tofu (or smoked if you prefer).
2 medium carrots, grated
1 inch (2.5cm) round of red cabbage, chopped
2 spring onions, finely chopped
2 sticks celery, sliced
4 broccoli florets, chopped
4 tablespoons French Dressing (p. 148)

1. Combine all the ingredients in a large bowl and season with black pepper.

TOFU AND AVOCADO DIP WITH CRUDITÉS

This delicious dip allows you to crunch away on a variety of raw vegetables. Serve it with seasonal crudités – carrots, cucumber, tomato, lettuce, celery, fennel, endive, Chinese leaves, mushrooms, peppers, cauliflower or broccoli.

8oz (200g) soft tofu
½ ripe avocado
2 dessertspoons cottage cheese
1 clove garlic, peeled
1 spring onion, roughly chopped
1 tablespoon parsley
a pinch of paprika
1 teaspoon tamari *or* soy sauce
black pepper to taste

1. Blend all the ingredients until smooth and serve with crudités.

ENERGY SOUP

This soup is blended raw and heated to serve. You can use the same method to invent other instant, high-energy soups.

4 medium carrots
6 broccoli florets
1 bunch watercress
12oz (300g) tofu
4 teaspoons Vecon/Marigold stock
1 dessertspoon tomato purée
1 teaspoon spices *or* herbs to taste
½ pint (300ml) skimmed *or* soya milk

1. Put all the ingredients in a blender and process well.
2. Serve cold or gently heated (do not boil) with oat cakes.

Dinners

FISH PIE

This is my favourite fish recipe. Make sure you ask for colouring-free smoked haddock. Smoked haddock never used to be bright yellow and the yellow dyes are not good for you anyway.

4oz (100g) combined white fish and colouring-free smoked haddock
¼oz (6g) butter
½ tablespoon wholemeal flour
2½fl oz (75ml) skimmed *or* soya milk
2½oz (60g) prawns
2oz (50g) mushrooms
½ teaspoon mixed herbs
black pepper to taste
12oz (300g) mashed potato
1 tablespoon sesame seeds

1. Steam the fish for 15 minutes.
2. Heat the butter in a pan, stir in the flour, then gradually beat in the milk, to make a white sauce.
3. Combine the fish, white sauce, prawns, mushrooms and herbs.
4. Place in an oven-proof dish and top with the mashed potato.
5. Sprinkle with the sesame seeds.
6. Bake for 30 minutes at 200°C/400°F/gas mark 6.

CHILLI

This wonderful dish has fooled many a hardy meat-eater. Turkey mince can be substituted if you prefer. It can also be prepared in double quantity and frozen.

1 small onion, peeled and sliced
2 cloves garlic, peeled and crushed
½ green pepper, sliced
1 tablespoon olive oil
½ teaspoon chilli powder
1 teaspoon paprika
1 teaspoon ground cumin
1 teaspoon ground coriander
3oz (75g) soya mince or 8oz (200g) Quorn mince
½ × 9oz (225g) can tomatoes, chopped
1 tablespoon tomato purée
½ small can kidney beans

1. Steam-fry the onion, garlic and pepper in oil with the chilli powder, paprika, cumin and coriander.
2. Add the soya mince or Quorn and stir for two minutes.
3. Add the tomatoes, tomato purée and kidney beans. Mix well and leave to simmer for at least 30 minutes, stirring occasionally to prevent the bottom from burning. If the mixture becomes too thick, add a little water.

STEAM-FRIED VEGETABLES WITH . . .

This dish can be prepared with a variety of ingredients and seasonings. Choose one of the protein-rich foods, and one of the sauces, to combine with vegetables.

FOR THE PROTEIN:
12oz (300g) tofu, cubed
or 4oz (100g) chicken, cubed
or 12oz (300g) tempeh, cubed
or 6oz (150g) filleted fish, cubed

FOR THE SAUCE:
Thai: fresh coriander, green curry paste and a dash of coconut milk
Chinese: tamari (or soy sauce), ginger and garlic
Mexican: watered-down Mexican spice sauce (but check ingredients)
Mediterranean: tomatoes with mixed herbs
Indian: tomatoes with coriander, cumin and chilli powder

FOR THE VEGETABLES:
Choose from: spring onions, garlic, carrots, broccoli, courgettes, cauliflower, sugar snap peas, runner beans, water chestnuts, mushrooms, bean sprouts, peppers, bamboo shoots, etc.

1. Steam-fry some onion and garlic in your chosen sauce, add your protein-rich food and steam-fry until cooked.
2. Add a little water and your chosen vegetables. Simmer until the vegetables are cooked but still crunchy, and serve.

ROASTED VEGETABLES WITH QUINOA AND HARISSA

With its high protein content, quinoa is a remarkable food. In this dish, it is perfectly complemented by the roasted vegetables. The spicy sauce is a variation on the North African harissa.

10 cherry tomatoes
1 medium carrot, sliced
1 medium courgette, diced
1 red pepper, sliced
4 button mushrooms
1 medium onion, cut into 8
2 dessertspoons olive oil
8oz (200g) quinoa
1½ pints (860ml) water

FOR THE HARISSA:
2 tinned plum tomatoes
¼ teaspoon cayenne pepper
1 teaspoon ground cumin
1 teaspoon ground coriander
1 clove garlic
a dash of vinegar

1. Place all the vegetables on a baking tray and lightly drizzle with olive oil.
2. Bake in a preheated oven, at 180°C/350°F/gas mark 4 for 50 minutes. Remove twice during cooking and shake tray to turn and recoat vegetables.
3. Meanwhile, rinse the quinoa very well under cold, running water.
4. Put it in a saucepan with the water, bring to the boil, cover and simmer for 13 minutes or until the water has boiled away.
5. Blend the harissa ingredients to form a paste. Add a dash of vinegar if the paste is too stiff.
6. Serve a mound of quinoa topped with vegetables and a little harissa on the side.

GRILLED BURGERS*

Here is a home-made, vegetarian alternative to the hamburger! Many supermarkets now stock good ready-made vegetarian burgers and sausages. Choose ones without hydrogenated fat or additives.

12oz (300g) tofu, mashed
4 tablespoons soy sauce
1 medium carrot, grated
1 garlic clove, peeled and crushed
1 small spring onion, chopped
2 slices wholegrain rye bread, toasted and crumbed
1 tablespoon tomato purée
1 medium free-range egg
salt and pepper to taste
1 tablespoon fresh coriander, chopped
1 tablespoon olive oil

1. Mix the tofu and soy sauce in a bowl, leave for 20 minutes, then squeeze out and discard any excess moisture.
2. Mix all the ingredients, except the oil, in a bowl and form into four burgers. Chill for 20 minutes.
3. Lightly brush the burgers with oil and grill under a medium grill for 15 minutes, turning frequently.
4. Serve between two slices of rye bread with sliced tomato and lettuce.

* Courtesy of Cauldron foods

THAI BAKED COD

Thai seasoning is subtle and delicious. You can use any white fish – it doesn't have to be cod. The dish is even better if the fish is left to marinate in the sauce for a few hours before cooking. It goes very well with Crunchy Thai Salad (p.146).

2 medium cod fillets
juice and grated zest of 1 lime
½ inch (1 cm) ginger root, grated
1 stick lemon grass, sliced
2 cloves garlic, peeled and crushed
1 teaspoon tamari *or* soy sauce
1 fresh chilli, finely chopped

1. In a mug, blend the lime juice, lime zest, grated ginger, lemon grass, crushed garlic, tamari or soy sauce and chilli. (Beware – when you chop the chilli, wash your hands immediately.)
2. Rinse the cod fillets and place them in a baking dish.
3. Pour over the lime mixture, turning the fish so it is well coated. Ideally, leave to marinate for at least an hour or overnight.
4. Cover with a lid or tin foil and bake in a preheated oven, at 200°C/400°F/gas mark 6, for 20 minutes (or until cooked, which will depend on the thickness of the fish).

GRILLED PESTO CHICKEN

This dish has a wonderful Mediterranean taste and goes very well with Tomato and Broccoli Salad (p. 147).

2 medium chicken breasts, rinsed
1 dessertspoon pesto

1. Slice the rinsed chicken breasts crossway and spread half the pesto inside
2. Spread the remaining pesto on top of the chicken and grill for 25 minutes (or until cooked, which will depend on the thickness of the chicken).

DAHL (LENTIL CURRY)

This dish – a favourite of mine – is a variation on a recipe given to me by a lady from Goa. Despite the lentils, it always goes down well with meat-eaters. Leftovers can be frozen or eaten with a baked potato for lunch the following day.

11oz (275g) orange lentils
1¾ (1 litre) pint water
1 medium onion, peeled and chopped
4 cloves garlic, peeled and chopped
1 heaped teaspoon curry powder
1 teaspoon Vecon *or* Marigold stock
1 × 16oz (400g) can tomatoes

1. Rinse the lentils well in cold, running water until the water runs clear.
2. Place in a saucepan with the water, onion and garlic.
3. Bring to the boil and simmer for 20 minutes.
4. Add the curry powder, stock paste/powder and tomatoes and stir well. Cover and leave to simmer for a further 30 minutes, stirring occasionally to make sure the bottom does not burn. If it starts to get too thick, add a little water or if it seems too watery, leave uncovered.

COLESLAW

Cabbages are packed with vitamins and minerals. So are carrots (high in vitamin A) and onions (high in sulphur–containing amino acids, which help to remove toxins from the body).

8oz (200g) red or white cabbage
4oz (100g) carrots
½ small onion
1 tablespoon low-fat mayonnaise
1 tablespoon very low-fat yoghurt
½ tablespoon skimmed milk

1. Finely chop the cabbage, carrots and onion.
2. Mix all the ingredients together in a bowl, and serve.

CARROT SOUP IN THE RAW

Ever had a hot, raw soup? This soup is made cold and heated gently, keeping all the vitamin and mineral content intact. It's also full of fibre. Don't overheat it.

8oz (200g) carrots
1½ oz (35g) ground almonds
5fl oz (150ml) skimmed *or* soya milk
1 teaspoon vegetable stock
½ teaspoon mixed herbs

1. Place the carrots in a food processor and blend to a purée.
2. Add other ingredients and process until mixed.
3. Warm very gently in a pan.

CRUNCHY THAI SALAD

This is a variation on one of the most popular 'street food' dishes in Thailand, where it is made to order – in a mortar and pestle – never in advance. It originally comes from the Northeast of the country, but is now available in your own kitchen!

¼ medium white cabbage, finely shredded
8 runner beans, chopped
1 medium tomato, chopped
1 chilli, very finely chopped
juice of 2 limes
1 dessertspoon fish sauce
1 dessertspoon apple juice
1 handful unsalted peanuts, roughly crushed

1. Combine all the ingredients in a large bowl and toss well. If you are not keen on hot food, leave out the chilli, or take care not to eat the pieces once they have flavoured the salad.

GREEN SALAD

This simple green salad is a good accompaniment to any meal.

½ cos or other lettuce, roughly torn
¼ bulb of fennel, sliced
4 broccoli florets, chopped
¼ cucumber, chopped
2 sticks celery, sliced
1 tablespoon French Dressing (p. 148)

1. Combine all the ingredients and toss with the French dressing.

WATERCRESS SALAD

Watercress is rich in iron and vitamin A and is delicious in salad.

½ bunch watercress
½ little gem lettuce, sliced
¼ cucumber, sliced
½ green pepper, chopped
1 handful alfalfa sprouts
1 tablespoon French Dressing (p.148)

1. Combine all the ingredients and toss with the French dressing.

MEDITERRANEAN TOMATO AND BROCCOLI SALAD

10 – 15 cherry tomatoes, halved
6 medium broccoli florets, chopped
6 large, fresh basil leaves, roughly torn
1 dessertspoon olive oil
2 teaspoons balsamic vinegar
black pepper to taste

1. Toss all the ingredients together and serve.

FRENCH DRESSING

This standard French dressing can be jazzed up by adding fresh and dried herbs. Also experiment with other oils such as cold-pressed sesame oil or flax oil which contains EFAs. Use as little dressing as possible on salads.

3 tablespoons extra-virgin olive oil
1 tablespoon Essential Balance *or* Udo's Choice (see Useful Addresses)
2 tablespoons cider vinegar
1 tablespoon French mustard
1 clove garlic, peeled and crushed

1. Put all the ingredients in a screw-top jar and shake vigorously. Any extra dressing can be stored in the bottle in the fridge.

TAHINI DRESSING

Tahini is crushed sesame seeds and their oil – it makes a dressing thicker and creamier.

EITHER:
2 tablespoons French Dressing (see above)
1 tablespoon tahini

OR:
1 tablespoon Honey and Mustard Dressing (from the supermarket)
1 tablespoon Essential Balance *or* Udo's Choice
1 tablespoon tahini
a squeeze of lemon juice

1. Put all the ingredients in a screw-top jar and shake vigorously. Any extra dressing can be stored in the bottle in the fridge.

Desserts

APRICOT WHISK

This dessert tastes even better than it looks. Using dried apricots, rich in micronutrients, it can be made all year round.

4 oz (100 g) dried *or* fresh apricots
¼ teaspoon natural vanilla essence
5oz (125g) low-fat natural yoghurt
3oz (75g) cottage cheese
1 egg white

1. Stew the apricots until soft. (Soak overnight, if using dried apricots.)
2. Blend in a processor, adding the vanilla essence, yoghurt and cottage cheese.
3. Whisk the egg white until stiff and fold into the apricot mixture.
4. Place in a bowl, or individual glasses, and chill before serving.

FRESH FRUIT SALAD

Adding one or two interesting fruits improves a fruit salad enormously. For example, try mango, kiwi, fresh lychees, strawberries, fresh dates or melon.

1lb (400g) mixed fruits
1oz (25g) dried apricots (soaked overnight)
4 tablespoons natural yoghurt

1. Cut the fruit into cubes.
2. Stew the apricots and liquidise, adding enough water to make a pourable sauce.
3. Pour the cooled sauce and natural yoghurt over the fresh fruit, and serve.

RASPBERRY SURPRISE

This fruit fool is also delicious made with strawberries or blackcurrants.

8oz (200g) raspberries (fresh, *or* frozen and thawed)
4oz (100g) low-fat fromage frais
1–2 teaspoons runny honey
handful of fresh mint leaves.

1. Blend raspberries, fromage frais and honey.
2. Pour into individual serving dishes. Garnish with a sprig of mint.

HUNZA APRICOTS WITH CASHEW CREAM

4oz (100g) Hunza apricots
1oz (25g) whole hazelnuts
3oz (75g) cashew nuts

1. Soak the apricots in boiling water.
2. When soft remove the stones and replace each one with a whole hazelnut.
3. Grind the cashews in a blender until fine. Slowly trickle in water until you have a creamy consistency.
4. Serve the apricots with the cashew cream in a sundae glass.

RHUBARB AND BLACKCURRANT PIE

If you like rhubarb you'll love the combination of rhubarb and blackcurrant in this pie. You can use any seasonal fruits.

8oz (200g) rhubarb
4oz (100g) blackcurrants
¼ teaspoon ground ginger
4oz (100g) cottage cheese
3fl oz (75ml) skimmed milk
½ tablespoon honey
2 tablespoons ground almonds

1. Stew the rhubarb and blackcurrants until soft in a small amount of water.
2 Mix in ginger and put in ovenproof dish.
3 Mix cottage cheese, milk and honey together thoroughly.
4 Cover fruit with curd cheese mixture.
5 Sprinkle with almonds and lightly toast under a hot grill.

FRUIT KEBABS

1 green apple
1 red apple
1 banana
a little lemon juice
1 orange
6 black grapes
8oz (200g) natural yoghurt
1 teaspoon honey

1. Cube the apples and banana and coat with a little lemon juice to prevent them from going brown.
2. Peel the orange, removing all the pith, and cut into chunks. Halve the grapes and remove the pips.
3. Put the fruit onto skewers and grill under a high grill or on a barbecue.
4. Blend the yoghurt with the honey and use as a dipping sauce.

RASPBERRY SORBET

There are many variations on this theme, which allow you to pick fruit in season, freeze it and use it whenever you want. Just think – raspberries and strawberries all year round!

1 banana, chopped into ½ inch (1cm) lengths
8oz (200g) frozen raspberries
4 tablespoons natural yoghurt

1. Freeze the banana chunks.
2. Remove the bananas and raspberries from the freezer and allow to partially thaw – about five minutes.
3. Blend the fruit with the yoghurt in a food processor and serve immediately.

PEACH AND CAROB CREAMS*

4 oz (100g) tofu
½ × 16oz (400g) can peaches in juice
3 tablespoons honey
½ medium banana
1 teaspoon agar agar
2 teaspoons carob powder
1 small carob bar, grated

1. Liquidise the tofu, the peaches and their juice, the honey and banana.
2. Blend 5fl oz (150ml) water with the agar agar and carob powder in a small saucepan and bring to the boil, stirring constantly. Pour into the mixture in the liquidiser and blend until smooth.
3. Transfer to one large or four individual dishes and chill.
4. Decorate with the grated carob.

*Courtesy of Cauldron foods

REFERENCES

Part 1

1 Wolever, T., *The Glycaemic Index*.

2 Rankins, J., 'Glycemic Index and Exercise metabolism', *Gatorade Sports Sci Ins Sport Sci Exchange*, 10(1) (1997).

3 Heaton, K. et al, 'Particle size of wheat, maize and oat test meals: effects on plasma glucose and insulin responses and on the rate of starch digestion in vitro', *Am. J. Clin. Nutr.* 47:675–82 (1988).

4 Wunderlich, R., *Sugar and Your Health*, Good Health Publications, Florida (1982).

5 Davies, S., 'Zinc, Nutrition and Health' chapter in *1984/5 Yearbook of Nutritional Medicine* (1985).

6 Davies, S. et al., 'Age-related decreases in chromium levels in 51,665 hair, sweat and serum samples from 40,872 patients – implications for the prevention of cardiovascular disease and type II diabetes mellitus', *Metabolism*, 46(5):1–4 (1997).

7 Bensky et al., 'Chinese Herbal medicine', *Materia Medica*, Eastland Press (1986).

8 Brekham, I. & Dardymov, I., 'Pharmacological Investigation of Glycosides from Ginseng and Eleutherococcus', Lloydia, 32:46–51 (1969).
Brekham, I. & Dardymov, I., 'New Substances of Plant Origin which Increase Nonspecific Resistance', *Annual Review of Pharmacology*, 9:419–30 (1969).

Part 2

1 Cox, I.M. et al., 'Red blood cell magnesium and chronic fatigue syndrome', *Lancet*, 337:757–60 (1991).

Ahlborg, L.G. et al., 'Effect of potassium-magnesium aspartate on the capacity for prolonged exercise in man', *Acta Physiologica Scandinavia*, 74:238–45 (1969).

Hicks, J.T., 'Treatment of fatigue in general practice: a double blind study', *Clin. Med.*, 85–90 (1964).

Shaw, D.L., 'Management of fatigue: a physiologic approach', *Am. J. Med. Sci.*, 43:758–69 (1962).

2 Rigden, S. et al., 'Management of chronic fatigue symptoms by tailored nutritional intervention using a program designed to support hepatic detoxification', Health Comm Inc.

3 Rigden, S. et al., 'Evaluation of the effect of a modified entero-hepatic resuscitation program in chronic fatigue syndrome patients', Functional Medicine Research Center (March 1997).

Part 3

1 Silverberg, D.S., 'Non-pharmacological treatment of hypertension', *J. Hypertens. Suppl.*, 8(4):521–26 (Sept. 1990).

2 Hammond, C.E., 'Some preliminary findings on physical complaints from a prospective study of 1,064,004 men and women', *Am. J. Public Health*, 54:11–23 (1964).

3 Delmonte, M.M., 'Physiological concomitants of meditation practice', *Int. J. of Psychosomatics*, 31:23 (1984).

4 Keicolt-Glaser, J.K. et al., 'Modulation of cellular immunity in medical students', *J. of Behavioural Medicine*, 9:5 (1986).

5 Delmonte, M.M., 'Meditation as a clinical intervention strategy: a brief review', *Int. J. of Psychosomatics*, 31 (1984).

Part 4

1 Popper, H. & Steigmann, F., *Am. Med. Assoc.*, 123:1108–114 (1943).

Recommended Reading

Part 1

The GI Factor, Anthony Leeds, Jennie Brand Miller, Kaye Foster-Powell and Stephen Colagiuri, Hodder & Stoughton (1996)
Enter The Zone, Barry Sears PhD, Regan Books (1995)
The Fatburner Diet, Patrick Holford, Piatkus (1999)

Part 2

Improve Your Digestion, Patrick Holford, Piatkus (2009)
Detoxification and Healing, Sidney MacDonald Baker MD, Keats Publishing (1997)
The 20-Day Rejuvenation Diet Programme, Jeffrey Bland PhD, Keats Publishing (1997)

Part 3

Master Level Exercise – Psychocalisthenics, Oscar Ichazo, Sequoia Press (1993)
Meditate Swami Muktananda, State University of New York Press (1991)
What's On My Mind? Swami Anantananda, SYDA (1996)
Timeshifting Stephen Rechtschaffen, Rider Books (1996)

USEFUL ADDRESSES

The Arica Institute, founded by Oscar Ichazo, offers one-day trainings in the 'Doors of Compensation®'. Visit www.arica.org/trainings/schedule.cfm for details of trainings worldwide. In the US contact the Arica Institute Inc., PO Box 645, Kent, CT 06757-0645, USA. Tel: 860 927 1006 or email info@arica.org.

Essential Oil Blends containing a combination of cold-pressed seed oils are becoming more widely available. The best two products are LipoCare from BioCare, Tel: +44 (0) 121 433 3727 or visit www.biocare.co.uk, or Udo's Choice, distributed by Savant Distribution Limited, Quarry House, Clayton Wood Close, Leeds, LS16 6QE. Tel: +44 (0) 113 388 5230.

BioCare produce a wide range of supplements. They also supply Low GL Get Up & Go, Chill Food and Awake Food. Tel: +44 (0) 121 433 3727 or visit www.biocare.co.uk.

The Institute for Optimum Nutrition offers a three-year foundation degree course in nutritional therapy that includes training in the optimum nutrition approach to mental health. There is a clinic, a list of nutrition practitioners across the UK, an information service and a quarterly journal – *Optimum Nutrition*. Contact ION at Avalon House, 72 Lower Mortlake Road, Richmond TW9 2JY, Tel: +44 (0) 20 8614 7800 or visit www.ion.ac.uk.

Laboratory Tests can be undertaken through qualified clinical nutritionists and doctors. (To find a clinical nutritionist see below.)

Meditation There are a number of different approaches and courses available. Two that have received good feedback are the courses offered by Siddha Yoga Centre, The Amadeus Centre, 50 Shirland Road, Little Venice, London W9 2JA, visit www.syduk.org, and courses offered by the London Buddhist Centre at 51 Roman Road, London E2 0HU. Tel: +44 (0) 208 981 1225 or visit www.lbc.org.uk. Both groups have regional networks.

Nutrition Consultation To find a nutritionist in your area, visit www.patrickholford.com and click on 'Advice' and then 'Find a Nutritionist'. If there is no-one nearby, you can always do an online assessment – see below.

Online 100% Health Programme How healthy are you? Find out with our FREE health check and comprehensive, personalised 100% Health Programme giving you a personalised action plan, including diet and supplements. Visit www.patrickholford.com.

Psychocalisthenics is an excellent exercise system that takes less than twenty minutes a day, and develops strength, suppleness and stamina and generates vital energy. The best way to learn it is to do the Psychocalisthenics Training. See www.patrickholford.com ('events') for details and to order the book *Master Level Exercise: Psychocalisthenics* and the Psychocalisthenics CD and DVD. For further information please see www.pcals.com.

Solgar produce an extensive range of supplements available through health food shops. For your nearest stockist, contact Solgar Vitamins Ltd, Beggars Lane, Aldbury, Tring, Herts HP23 5PT, visit www.solgar.co.uk.

INDEX

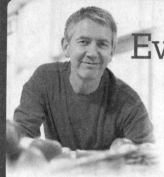

How 100% Healthy are you?

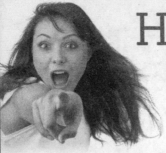

"I thought I was a healthy person. I did the online report. I feel absolutely fantastic. It's changed my life. It's amazing." Karen S

Karen before 36%

Karen after 86%

D	C	B	A
NOT GOOD	AVERAGE	REASONABLY HEALTHY	HEALTHY

YOU CAN wake up full of energy, with a clear mind and balanced mood, never gain weight and stay disease free. Having worked with over 60,000 people We know what changes are going to most rapidly transform how you feel. The **100% Health Programme** is the most comprehensive and genuinely effective way of taking a step towards 100% health.

Your **FREE Health Check** is the first step to receiving your **100% Health Programme** (£24.95), the ultimate on-line personal health profile, that shows you exactly what your perfect diet and daily supplement programme is, and which simple lifestyle changes will make the biggest difference.

You receive:

- ✔ A full Set of Results on your body systems and processes
- ✔ In-depth Report on you & your health
- ✔ Your Perfect Recipes and Menu Plan
- ✔ Your own Library of Special Reports
- ✔ Full Lifestyle Analysis inc:
  • Exercise • Stress • Sleep • Pollution
- ✔ Your Action Plan & Personal Supplement Programme;
- ✔ PLUS optional weekly support and guidance from Patrick;
- ✔ Free Reassessment to chart your progress, month by month
- ✔ Your questions answered by Patrick himself, plus all the benefits of membership

BEGIN YOUR **FREE** HEALTH CHECKUP NOW
Go to **www.patrickholford.com**

100%Health®
Weekend Intensive

The workshop that works.

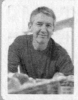